HUMAN EXPERIMENTATION

Human Experimentation

Methodologic issues
fundamental to clinical trials

by

TON J. CLEOPHAS, M.D., Ph.D

President -elect American College of Angiology,
F.A.C.A.,
Co-chairman basic module Medical Statistics
European Diploma of Pharmaceutical Medicine.
c/o Albert Schweitzer Hospital Dordrecht, Netherlands.

Kluwer Academic Publishers

Dordrecht / Boston / London

A C.I.P. Catalogue record for this book is available from the Library of Congress.

ISBN 0-7923-5827-9

Published by Kluwer Academic Publishers,
P.O. Box 17, 3300 AA Dordrecht, The Netherlands.

Sold and distributed in North, Central and South America
by Kluwer Academic Publishers,
101 Philip Drive, Norwell, MA 02061, U.S.A.

In all other countries, sold and distributed
by Kluwer Academic Publishers,
P.O. Box 322, 3300 AH Dordrecht, The Netherlands.

Printed on acid-free paper

Printed in the Netherlands

TABLE OF CONTENTS

FOREWORD   ix

PREFACE   xi

CHAPTER 1   PLACEBOS   1

1.1   Introduction   1
1.2   Ethical problems with placebo-controlled trials   1
1.3   Benefits of placebo-controlled trials   2
1.4   Technical problems with placebo-controlled trials   3
1.5   Conclusions   4

CHAPTER 2   FUNDAMENTAL ISSUES OF
             CHOOSING THE RIGHT TYPE OF TRIAL   7

2.1   Introduction   7
2.2   Ethical problems   8
2.3   Costs   8
2.4   Sample size   9
2.5   Between-subject variability of symptoms   9
2.6   Physical carryover effects   10
2.7   Time effects   10
2.8   Correlation between treatment modalities   11
2.9   Conclusions and examples   12

CHAPTER 3   LACK OF REAL SCIENCE OF
             SYMPTOM-BASED CARE   15

3.1   Introduction   15
3.2   Methods   17
3.3   Study selection and data extraction   17
3.4   Data synthesis   17
3.5   Discussion   20

CHAPTER 4   CARRYOVER EFFECTS IN CLINICAL RESEARCH   25

4.1   Introduction   25
4.2   Dose response and dose titration studies   26
4.3   Studies with duplicate standard deviations   28
4.4   Open evaluations studies   29
4.5   Cross-over studies   30
4.6   Self-controlled Studies   32
4.7   Parallel-group studies   33
4.8   Studies with subjective variables   33
4.9   Discussion   35

**CHAPTER 5   CRITICISM OF NEGATIVE STUDIES DUE TO
                NEGATIVE CORRELATIONS   37**

5.1   Introduction   37
5.2   Levels of correlation and sensitivity of testing   38
5.3   A simple test to check a posteriori whether the cause
       of a negative result is its level of correlation   39
5.4   Review of published crossover studies with
       a presumably negative correlation   40
5.5   Review of published crossover studies with
       a presumably positive correlation   42
5.6   Conclusions and recommendations   44
5.7   Conclusions   46

**CHAPTER 6   BETWEEN-GROUP DISPARITIES
                IN DRUG RESPONSE   48**

6.1   Introduction   48
6.2   Statistical model   49
6.3   Hypothetical examples, power analysis   52
6.4   Discussion   55

CHAPTER 7   SPECIFIC PROBLEMS WITH TRIALS OF
             CHRONIC DISEASES   57

7.1   Introduction   57
7.2   Published clinical trials   58
7.3   Strengths and weaknesses of the two designs   58
7.4   Stage of study and the type of trial   61
7.5   More recent statistical papers on the subject   62
7.6   Conclusions   62

CHAPTER 8   CLINICAL TRIALS WITH NEW ENDPOINTS   66

8.1   Introduction   66
8.2   Subjective endpoints   67
8.3   New ethical priorities   67
8.4   Human touch rather than scientific rigor   68
8.5   Little emphasis on informed consent   69
8.6   Self-controlled rather than parallel-group designs   69
8.7   Conclusions   71

CHAPTER 9   LINEAR SCALE ASSESSMENT OF RELEVANT
             DOMAINS OF QUALITY OF LIFE - an example   73

9.1   Introduction   73
9.2   Patients and methods   74
9.3   Results   76
9.4   Discussion   76

CHAPTER 10   ITEM RESPONSE MODELING AND
             QUALITY OF LIFE   81

10.1 Introduction   81
10.2 Methods   82
10.3 Results   83
10.4 Discussion   86

**CHAPTER 11 IS SELECTIVE REPORTING
              OF WELL-DESIGNED RESEARCH
              UNETHICAL AS WELL AS UNSCIENTIFIC ?**   90

11.1 Introduction   91
11.2 Arguments against reporting "negative" studies   91
11.3 Arguments in favor of reporting "negative" studies   93
11.4 How progress of science was made in the past   94
11.5 Today the progress of science is faster, new rules are required 95
11.6 Suggestions for a balanced approach
       to the problem of selective reporting   96
11.7 Conclusions   97

**CHAPTER 12 INFORMED CONSENT UNDER SCRUTINY,
              SUGGESTIONS FOR IMPROVEMENT**   99

12.1 Introduction   100
12.2 Ethical difficulties with the informed consent principle   100
12.3 Ethical difficulties with the informed consent process   102
12.4 Example of a flawed consent information form
       of a double-blind parallel-group study   103
12.5 Suggestions for improvement of the informed consent procedure 105
12.6 Conclusion   105

FOREWORD

The last decades have witnessed a dramatic and welcome improvement in the methods of drug evaluation and therefore our ability to use biological or pharmaceutical agents which benefit to risk ratio has been better assessed.

While these changes have had an immense impact on the professional day to day lives of all of those involved in human experimentation, there are still growing expectations for education information and reflections in this more demanding environment.

In this respect, the book by T.J. Cleophas displays several original aspects. Each chapter is derived from personal papers published over the last decade. It not only covers methodological issues but also discusses ethical, clinical and costs implications. It also provides non classical recommendations to be taken into account by clinical pharmacologists and clinicians when choosing the appropriate type of clinical trial and new models to statisticians when analysing those trials, all supported by substantial references.

The author dares to question some dogma such as the use of placebo controlled studies or the systematic use of objective outcomes and integrates a philosophical approach into the consideration of scientific truths. He leads the reader to think about not only the methods but also the purposes of clinical experimentation.

Let us thank T.J. Cleophas for challenging conventional rules and proposing alternatives that are likely to bring progress into the methodologies of clinical trials.

J.Ph. Santoni M.D.
Medical & Regulatory
Affairs Director Pharmacology,
Synthelabo Group,
Nanterre, France

J.P. Boissel M.D.
Professor of Clinical pharmacology
Claude Bernard
Université,
Lyon, France

PREFACE

Since the early fifties when the first randomized controlled trials were published, this scientific method has entered an era of continuous improvement, and has gradually become accepted as the most effective way of determining the relative efficacy and toxicity of new treatments. Even so, trials are sometimes inadequate, and widespread problems exist in the published literature of clinical trials. The current book tries to address such inadequacies and problems, and to provide solutions for that purpose. The data of this book are obtained from the literature as well as from the author's own experience with clinical trials. The book is intended not only for those involved in clinical research, but also for those who wish to apply research evidence to individual patients.

ACKNOWLEDGMENTS

The author is indebted to Dr Jan van der Meulen, and Dr Piet Tavenier of the Merwede Hospital Dordrecht, Netherlands, and Dr Menco G. Niemeyer of the Martini Hospital Groningen, Netherlands, for invaluable support in preparing this manuscript. Also I wish to thank Prof. Dr Rob B. Kalmansohn of the University of California in Los Angeles at UCLA, USA, Dr Aeilko H. Zwinderman of Leiden University, Netherlands, and Ruudje C. Cleophas of Rotterdam University Law School, Netherlands, for helpful comments and criticisms.

CHAPTER 1

PLACEBOS

The topic of placebos in clinical research has been recently addressed in general journals, and is relevant to a clinical pharmacologists' readership as well. We try to give an overview of benefits as well as problems of this methodology. Although the use of placebo in drug development is frequently absolutely essential, important ethical and technical problems are generally involved. We conclude that the placebo-controlled trial although methodologically pure may sometimes cause too much difficulties in the clinical setting.

1.1 Introduction

The topic of placebos in clinical research has been recently addressed in important general journals such as the Journal of the American Medical Association [1], the Lancet [2], the British Medical Journal [3], and the New England Journal of Medicine [4]. Turner *et al.* [1] noted that the placebo response in placebo-controlled trials involves rather complex phenomena including not only psychological placebo effects but also patient expectations of being helped and characteristics of the treatment situation that influence patients to report improvement. Kleijnen *et al.* [2] assume that placebos do not adequately control for placebo effects because of unadjusted patient expectations in the course of a trial. Ernst and Resch [3] stress that the true and the perceived placebo effect may be largely different. There is, thus, growing awareness that the placebo-controlled trial is not a simple method to determine the true treatment effect of a test compound as compared to placebo. We should add that the use of placebo in patients unlike healthy subjects frequently raises ethical problems, particularly in conditions with an established treatment modality at hand [4].

1.2 Ethical problems with placebo-controlled trials

In spite of these quarrels the use of placebo controls is extremely common in current clinical research. Also, for the purpose of statistical power patients are frequently treated for long periods of time, for example, in the many phase III mortality studies in patients with myocardial infarction: 41.4 months in SOLVD I [5], 37 months in SOLVD II [6], 42 months in SAVE [7], and 25 months in MDPIT [8]. An additional point is that quite large numbers of patients are generally involved. Lau *et al.* [8] calculated that 10,000 patients would be needed for demonstrating whether a treatment would reduce mortality from heart disease by 5%, which means with a statistically significant result at p = 0.05. Even then there is a chance of 5% that the established difference is based on an error. GISSI [10] and ISIS IV [11] included, therefore, not less than 20,000 and 60,000 patients. Finally, millions of dollars are required for the execution of this kind of placebo-controlled mega-trials[12], which in itself is in striking contrast with the current context of relative scarcity that even in the Western world is starting to characterize health care.

The ethicist Immanuel Kant [13] emphasizes the primacy of the test subject: human beings by virtue of their unique capacity of rational thought have an inherent dignity which makes them superior to animals. It implies that they should not be used as means to an end but rather as ends in themselves. The essence of this statement can be recognized in the first lines of the Declaration of Helsinki [14], which investigators worldwide are compliant with: "A physician shall act only in the patient's interest.". Strictly this principle seems to be inconsistent with the prescription of a placebo to a patient. This very principle is one of the reasons for oncologists to decide that in their specialty placebo-controlled trials are only acceptable for support care indications and not for the treatment of the disease. How do specialists other than oncologists justify the use of such trials for the latter purpose. On the one hand, it seems ethical to prove that the efficacy of a new treatment is not entirely based on a placebo effect. On the other hand, it may not be very ethical to do so by treating a group of diseased persons with a placebo throughout a trial. A placebo is definitely inappropriate in life-threatening conditions with a well-established effective, albeit imperfect, treatment modality available. In this situation the new treatment should be tested either against the standard treatment or in addition to the standard treatment. If this is not available, is it ethical to use a placebo then? Perhaps not always, for example, if we have strong arguments to believe that the new treatment is indeed better than placebo which in many phase III trials is definitely so. We should add that in clinical medicine it is far from uncommon to base decisions on beliefs rather than proven facts.

1.3   Benefits of placebo-controlled trials

The most important reasons for the initiation of placebo-controlled trials are the following. First, this type of trial which is purely experimental in nature provides the rigor which is required for the generation of the most reliable data. The clinical trial even though it has problems, is in fact an essential methodology in drug development. In many situations, use of a placebo is absolutely essential. The most classic examples of this are the Cast Trials [15-17]. For many years physicians had treated patients with antierythmic drugs in an effort to reduce mortality and were actually increasing mortality. Secondly, investigators often use the argument that the interest of the community at large is superior to the interest of a group of individuals, when arguing placebo-controlled testing of potentially important compounds. For example, Yusuf et al. [18], and Antman et al. [19] use this argument to justify the appropriateness of a placebo group in large, simple randomized trials such as ISIS [11] or VHeFT [20], particularly in the setting where the effectiveness of a putative treatment is unknown or, at least, unproven. We should add that the ability of a clinical trial subject to give truly consent to participate in those placebo-controlled studies has been extensively debated and confirmed by medical ethicists [21-24]. Thirdly, in countries such as the USA and England new pharmaceutical compounds may not be registered until placebo-controlled trials have provided sufficiently powerful data. The problem is that in the absence of a placebo group, clinical trials would contain only an active control. A trial comparing only two or more active treatments, in general, needs to be appreciably larger than a placebo-controlled study, since showing comparability between active treatments in the absence of a placebo is without meaning if a study is insufficiently powered to be able to detect a meaningful difference. If a new, "active" treatment is actually ineffective, then a placebo-controlled trial may minimize the number of individuals ultimately exposed to the ineffective treatment, arguably an ethically desirable outcome.

1.4 Technical problems with placebo-controlled trials

The evidence provided by placebo-controlled studies is, however, often considerably smaller than one might think. We should consider that a significant difference from placebo at p = 0.03, such as, for example, demonstrated in a subanalysis of the SOLVD study [25], means even so that a chance of 3% exists that the conclusion should have been "no difference" and a chance of only 70% exists that the conclusion "true difference" is justified. An additional point is the issue of little clinical relevance in spite of statistically significant findings. The above mentioned subanalysis for instance found no symptoms of angina pectoris in 85.3% of the patients on enalapril and in 82.5% of the patients on placebo [26]. In these kinds of situations one has to wonder about the clinical relevance of this small difference. This is particularly so when one considers that an active compound generally causes more side-effects than does a placebo. Finally, we have to consider the point of bias. Arguments have been raised that placebo-controlled trials and particularly the placebo-arm of such trials are especially vulnerable to bias [27]. Although intended to control for psychologic effects, they create an atmosphere of increased risks of such effects at the same time. For example, in clinical trials, as opposed to regular patient care, patients are generally highly compliant; their high compliance is an important reason for participating in the trial in the first place. They have a positive attitude towards the trial and anticipate personal benefit from it, a mechanism which in the psychology literature is known as the Hawthorne effect [28]. Also, they do not want to disappoint the investigators who are showing so much interest in them. These mechanisms may enhance the placebo response on the part of the participants. On the part of the investigators it may be extremely difficult to reveal the complete truth about the placebo, and the potential of a trial is usually "talked up". Furthermore, many phase III trials fail to obtain a written informed consent about the placebo. Therefore, the clinical trial, although intended to control for placebo effects, simultaneously creates an atmosphere of increased risks of such effects. An enhanced placebo effect can also occur as a consequence of carryover effect from the active treatment into the placebo treatment in crossover studies, and as a consequence of asymmetric placebo groups in parallel-group studies. Even if bias affects both of the treatment modalities similarly, the placebo data are likely to be damaged mostly. This is so, because placebo data are usually small, and small effects are more vulnerable to a fixed amount of bias than large effects are [29]. An additional problem of placebo-controlled studies is the fact that selected patients often refuse to comply with randomization. The remaining sample may be small and unrepresentative, and its relevance to the patients' population at large becomes difficult to judge. If in the end of these laborious efforts, including the recruitment of patients from different facilities, the results do not confirm the expectations of the investigators, one has to wonder if not we should use alternative methods for the evaluation of new treatment modalities more often.

1.5   Conclusions

In recent decades secondary prevention trials and mortality studies, particularly in patients with myocardial infarction, frequently made use of placebo controls. Some of us would say that, with life-threatening diseases, obtaining the greatest reliability about the effect of the treatment on death is more important than the ethical problems that may be involved in such an approach. Others, however, will not automatically agree on this point and will find that mortality as endpoint had better be replaced by morbidity more often, because the latter provides not only better sensitivity but also less ethical problems. Such endpoint may then be used as surrogate endpoint to estimate mortality. We should add that it is not necessarily the case that morbidity parallels mortality-witness the case with the phosphodiesterase inhibitor vasodilators in the treatment of congestive heart failure and hypertension where a variety of drugs improved exercise tolerance and even provided symptom benefit to patients at the expense of a significant increase in mortality [30].

Although placebo-controlled experimental research generally provides greater reliability than other forms of research, this very method sometimes causes major problems within the structure of a clinic where individual treatments of patients is priority. As a consequence of bias results may lose their scientific value. Case-control studies, retrospective and prospective cohort studies, and observational studies, although currently little used in the evaluation of a new drug or therapy, may be acceptable alternatives, that could be methods of choice, if the golden standard although methodologically pure, causes too much difficulties in the clinical setting.

Acknowledgement

The author is indebted to the editor and publisher of the British Journal of Clinical Pharmacology for granting permission to use part of a paper previously published in the journal (1997; 43: 219-21).

References

1. Turner JA, Deyo RA, Lieser JD, et al. The importance of placebo effects in pain treatment and research. JAMA 1994; 271: 1609-14.
2. Kleijnen J, de Craen AJM, Van Everdingen J, et al. Placebos in medicine. Placebo effect in double-blind clinical trials: a review of interactions with medications. Lancet 1994; 344: 1347-9.
3. Ernst E, Resch KL. Concept of true and perceived placebo effects. BMJ 1995; 311: 551-3.
4. Rothman KJ, Michels KB. The continuing unethical use of placebo controls. N Engl J Med 1994, 331: 394-8.
5. The SOLVD investigator. Effect of enalapril on survival in patients with reduced left ventricular ejection fractions and congestive heart failure. N Engl J Med 1991; 325: 293-302.
6. The SOLVD investigators. Effect of enalapril on mortality and the development of heart failure in asymptomatic patients with reduced left ventricular ejection fraction. N Engl J Med 1992; 327: 685-91.
7. Pfeffer MA, Braunwald E, Moyé L, et al. on behalf of the SAVE investigators. Effect of captopril on mortality and morbidity in patients with left ventricular dysfunction after myocardial infarction. Results of the Survival and Ventricular Enlargement Trial. N Engl J Med 1992; 327: 669-77.
8. The multicenter Diltiazem Post Infarction Trial Research Group. The effect of diltiazem on mortality and reinfarction after myocardial infarction. N Engl J Med 1988; 319: 385-92.
9. Lau J, Antman EM, Jimenez-Silva J, et al. Cumulative meta-analysis of therapeutic trials for myocardial infarction. N Engl J Med 1992; 327: 248-54.
10. Pfeffer MA. Angiotensin converting enzyme inhibition therapy following myocardial infarction: rationale for clinical trials. Herz 1991; 16: 278-82.
11. ISIS-4 Collaborative Group. Fourth International Study of Infarct Survival: protocol for a large simple study of the effects of oral mononitrate, of oral captopril, and of intravenous magnesium. Am J Cardiol 1991; 68: 87-100.
12. Doolittle RF. Biomedical research - the enormous costs of success. N Engl J Med 1991; 324: 1360-2.
13. Kant I. Kritik der Urteilskraft. Janecke. Leipzig, 1920.
14. World Medical Association. Declaration of Helsinki 1964, after revision adopted by the 41th World Medical Assembly, Hong Kong 1989.
15. The cardiac Suppression Trial II (CAST II) Investigators. Effect of the antiarrhythmic agent moricizine on survival after myocardial infarction. N Engl J Med 1992; 327: 227-33.
16. Echt DS, Liebson PB, Mitchell LB, et al. Mortality and morbidity in patients receiving encainide, flecainide, or placebo: the Cardiac Arrhythmia Suppression Trial. N Engl J Med 1991; 324: 781-8.
17. Greene HL, Roden DM, Katz RJ, et al. The Cardiac Arrhythmia Suppression Trial: first CAST... then CAST II. J Am Coll Cardiol 1992; 19: 804-8.
18. Yusuf S, Wittes J, Friedman L, et al. Overview of randomized trials in heart disease. Treatments following myocardial infarction. JAMA 1988; 260: 2088-93.
19. Antman EM, Lau J, Kupelnick B, et al. A comparison of results of meta-analyses of randomized controlled trials and recommendations of clinical experts: treatments for myocardial infarction. JAMA 1992; 268: 240-8.
20. Cohn JN, Archibald DG, Ziesche S, et al. Effect of vasodilator therapy on mortality in chronic congestive heart failure: results of a Veterans/Administration Cooperative Study. N Engl J Med 1986; 314: 547-52.
21. Brewin CR, Bradley C. Patients' preferences and randomised clinical trials. BMJ 1989; 299: 313-5.
22. Silverman WA, Altman DG. Patients' preferences and randomised trials. Lancet 1996; 347: 171-4.
23. Biros MH, Lewis RJ, Olson CM, et al. Informed consent in emergency research. JAMA 1995; 273: 1283-7.
24. Clayton EW, Steinberg KK, Khoury MJ, et al. Informed consent for genetic research. JAMA 1995; 274: 1786-92.
25. Yusuf S, Pepine CJ, Garces C, et al.: Effect of enalapril on myocardial infarction and unstable angina pectoris in patients with low ejection fractions. Lancet 1992; 340: 1173-8.
26. Cleophas TJM. The use of a placebo-control group in clinical trials. J Mol Med 1995; 73: 421-4.
27. Cleophas TJM. Clinical trials: design flaws associated with the use of a placebo. Am J Ther 1995; 3: 591-6.
28. Campbell JP, Maxey VA, Watson WA. Hawthorne effect: implications for prehospital research. Ann Emergency Med 1995; 26: 590-4.

29.Ernst E, Cleophas TJM, Turner JA, *et al.* The importance of placebo effects [letters]. JAMA 1995; 273: 283-4.

30.Packer M, Carver JR, Rodeheffer RJ, for the PROMISE Study Research group. Effect of oral milrinone on mortality in severe chronic heart failure. N Engl J Med 1991; 325: 1468-75.

CHAPTER 2

FUNDAMENTAL ISSUES OF CHOOSING
THE RIGHT TYPE OF TRIAL

Background. Relevant advantages and disadvantages of crossover/self-controlled and parallel-group studies are discussed.

Results. For ethicists crossovers are frequently less of a problem. Also, they may be less costly, and, in addition, statistically more powerful. If the treatments in a trial are curative, however, or if the variables are subjective, a parallel-group design is the right type of trial. In case of unstable disease, or a negative correlation in a treatment comparison, this is so.

Conclusions. Routinely including a set of rules prevents procedural biases and wrong study designs. The present study is a preliminary effort for the very effort of that.

2.1   Introduction

Só many unpredictable variables often play a role in clinical trials of medical treatments, that, by now, a trial without controls has become almost unconceivable. The following methods (Table I) are routinely used:

1. A single patient receives both a new therapy and a standard therapy or placebo (crossover or self-controlled design).
2. With every patient given a new therapy, a control patient is given a placebo or standard therapy (parallel-group design).

In the present paper we shall analyse relevant advantages and disadvantages of crossover/self-controlled and parallel-group studies. We will also discuss the clinical implications. Earlier reports have recognised elements of many of our points [1-3].

The choice of the right type of trial is a complex matter that has been considered the collective responsibility of clinical, laboratory, and statistical professionals.

The present overview tries to identify a set of rules that should help these professionals in doing their collaborative job. Some biases that enter trials are correctable. Procedural biases or wrong study designs, however, are not and require the investigators to start all over again [4]. Routinely including some kind of standard from the very start may help preventing this to happen. The present paper is a preliminary effort for the very purpose of that.

Table I.   Three basic types of controlled clinical trials
(combinations of the three or the use of additional groups or periods are possibilities)

1. Self-controlled Trial

	Period 1		Period 2	
	Treatment	Mean Efficacy	Treatment	Mean Efficacy
Single Group	Placebo	b	New Treatment	a

2. Crossover Trial

	Period 1		Period 2	
	Treatment	Mean Efficacy	Treatment	Mean Efficacy
Group A	New Treatment	a	Placebo	c
Group B	Placebo	b	New Treatment	d

3. Parallel-group Trial
A single period

	Treatment	Mean Efficacy
Group A	New Treatment	a
Group B	Placebo	b

2.2   Ethical problems

Ethicists generally do have less a problem with crossover/self-controlled than with parallelgroup designs[5]. In parallel-group studies a placebo or ineffective treatment is commonly used for long periods of time in a single group of patients. To do so may be ethically difficult to justify, particularly in patients with life threatening conditions, f.e., coronary artery disease. This is even more so if a well-established effective albeit not perfect treatment modality is already available. In this particular situation a placebo would seem definitely unethical, and a new treatment should be tested against the standard treatment instead of placebo either by a parallel or by a self-controlled design. Even then, however, because one treatment is frequently anticipated to be superior to the other, a self-controlled design would seem preferable since every test subject gets the same quantity of both the better and the worse.

2.3   Costs

Research should be cost effective, which implicates that a crossover/self-controlled design using one patient for the purpose of both test subject and control, should come the designer's mind in the first place. As we shall see there are some problems with self-controlled designs that may increase costs in such studies, however. F.e., crossovers and self-controlled studies take twice as much time as equivalent parallel-group studies. And time is supposed to be a major determinant of costs. A self-controlled design may even take substantially more time if a period of washout between two treatment periods is required. This means that the cost savings from a self-controlled/crossover design may be less substantial than one might think at first sight, as Brown has indicated [6]. On the other hand, however, another important determinant of costs of a trial is the number of tests at its completion. In a 20 subject vs 20 subject parallel-group study we have 40 tests in the end (20 vs 20 unpaired). In a 20 subject crossover we have equally 40 (20 vs 20 paired). So far, costs are equal. However, the paired comparison of the crossover is likely to provide more statistical power. The whole point of a crossover design is to use the generally positive correlation among observations for an individual to reduce the variability in a treatment comparison and to provide, thus, enhanced statistical power. The subject of correlation will be discussed in more detail in the section "correlation between treatment modalities". For now, we conclude that if we translate "cost effectivity" in terms of "statistical power for money" the crossover design will frequently be more cost effective.

2.4 Sample size

For one more reason the crossover design should come to the designer's mind in the first place. Parallel-group studies do need twice as many patients compared to equivalent self-controlled designs. This point may be decisive in rare diseases. Suppose, only 20 patients are available. A parallel-group study of 10 vs 10 subjects is difficult to stratify for symmetry of the covariates in the two groups, in the first place. Also, the unpaired comparison of 10 vs 10 in such a trial does have virtually no statistical power. Many crossovers in practice, however, include even less than 20 subjects. Also, they need not necessarily be stratified. It has been established that the paired within-subject comparison of a crossover [Table I: (a + d) minus (b + c); paired differences] can give strong evidence of a treatment effect even with 20 patients available. F.e., 41 crossovers in the Lancet and the New England Journal of Medicine in 1987 had to include only 8-32 subjects (mean value 22) [7] in order to be conclusive. The requirement of just a small group of patients is, of course, a blessing for any researcher, even the researcher of extremely common diseases. So, this is a strong point in favour of selfcontrolled designs, either for rare diseases or for the convenience of the investigators of any disease.

2.5 Between-subject variability of symptoms

For the study of cardiovascular diseases, f.e., hypertension and angina pectoris, properly designed crossover studies may be preferable to parallel-group studies. There is a considerable between-subject variability of symptoms in some of these conditions. Bias due to this factor is eliminated by the use of a crossover design [8-11]. However, the patients' symptoms in a trial is a variable of rather subjective nature. The problem with a crossover is that subjective variables are not in place because they are frequently biased by psychological carryover effect. F.e., if a patient is disappointed in the first period, he is likely to underestimate any effective treatment that comes next [11].

Therefore, for analysis of clinical symptoms a parallel-group design is required. This avoids the bias of underestimation or overestimation of a second treatment period. This is a bias that may be fatal to a trial.

2.6   Physical carryover effects

Designers of crossover and self-controlled studies should particularly be paying attention to the possibility of carryover effects. If the effect of the first treatment carries on into the next one, then it influences the response to the latter period. If for example treatment 1 consists of an effective antibiotic and treatment 2 is a placebo, then the patient will be cured after treatment 1 and the placebo effect will be as good as the real thing, since the patient is feeling well after treatment 1 [12]. Obviously, a crossover or selfcontrolled design should never be used where a treatment cures a disease. However, even with symptomatic therapies small curative effects can occur, f.e., wound healing by vasodilators. So, alertness is required. Just the fact that we have a purely symptomatic treatment under study does not implicate that we have no carry-over bias. Small carryover effects in a crossover study may be acceptable, since we have the possibility of testing it and correcting it [13-17]. We might imply that a presumably symptomatic treatment is suitable for a selfcontrolled design if other arguments are in favour of it as well.

2.7   Time effects

In phase 1-2 trials (Table II) short term effects of new treatments are studied in small groups of volunteers and/or patients, f.e., by means of dose response and dose titrations studies. Here, a crossover or self-controlled design is frequently used, so that a single subject can be tested more than once. For acute effects it may even be applied irrespective of the fact that a curative rather than symptomatic treatment is tested. In phase 3-4 trials things are different. Trials are considerably lengthy or long term. This means that acute diseases that have to be cured can only be studied through a parallel-group design. Some statisticians [18-24] and also the FDA [25] have even pointed out that in all phase 3-4 trials a parallel-group design should be applied and that there is basically no place for self-controlled or crossover designs here. The dilemma is that costs, thus, rise rapidly because we need twice as many test subjects and, in addition, that it is unethical to treat seriously ill patients for periods of months with placebo. It is our conviction therefore that in chronic stable diseases where cure is impossible, and where symptomatic treatment of a constant symptomatology is priority, phase 3-4 crossover trials do have an important place. All other advantages of self-controlled studies are involved, while the disadvantages are not relevant here.

Table II. Staging of clinical trials

	Who	Why	By whom
Fase 1	Normal subjects	Pharmacokinetics, Biologic effects	Clinical pharmacologists
Fase 2	Small group of patients	Dose titration, Therapeutic effects	Clinical pharmacologists
Fase 3	Larger group of patients	Safety, Efficacy	Clinical investigators
Fase 4	Large group of patients	Longterm effects, "Quality of life"	All physicians

2.8   Correlation between treatment modalities

In a comparison of two treatments the correlation between the two should be taken into account. F.e., in a trial the new treatment may be a slight modification of the standard or be equivalent to it with the addition of a new component. In these situations there is a positive correlation between the new and the standard treatment, which in case of a crossover assessment is enhanced by a generally small within-subject variability of symptoms. On the other hand, in trials with completely different treatments patients tend to fall apart into different populations: those who response to treatment A and those who do to treatment B. Patients with angina pectoris irresponsive to beta-blockers, generally do response either to calcium-antagonist or nitroglycerines. Also hypertension, Raynaud's syndrome, different types of cardiac arrhythmias are known to be conditions where a nonrespone to a particular compound is frequently associated with an excellent response to a completely different compound [26]. In such situations a strong negative correlation does exist. Figure 1 gives an example of how levels of correlation between treatment modalities influence these variances of paired differences opposedly. It can be seen that in the case of a negative correlation the standard deviation of the paired differences largely outnumbers the standard deviation of the positive correlation situation. This is the reason that finding a significant difference between two samples with the positive correlation is a lot easier than doing so with a negative. In the case of a negative correlation a crossover or selfcontrolled design is not appopriate due to lack of power. F.e., a crossover study of a betablocker and a diuretic in hypertension is, therefore, endangered of being biased by a type II error of finding no difference where there is one, because such trial would lack power due to the negative correlation between the two treatment options.

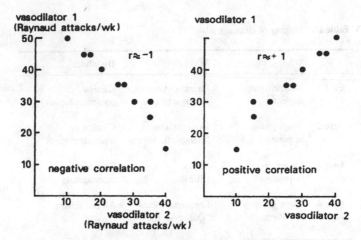

Figure 1. Two selfcontrolled studies with similar group means, n's and SD s,
but with largely different correlations.

	Study 1	Study 2
Individual Values Vasodilator 1	50, 45, 45, 40, 35, 35, 30, 30, 25, 15	15, 25, 30, 30, 35 35, 40, 45, 45, 50
Mean ± SD	**35 ± 10**	**35 ± 10**
Individual Values Vasodilator 2	10, 15, 15, 20, 25, 25, 30, 35, 35, 40	10, 15, 15, 20, 25 25, 30, 35, 35, 40
Mean ± SD	**25 ± 10**	**25 ± 10**
Paired Differences	40, 30, 30, 20, 10, 10, 0, -5, -10, -25	5, 10, 15, 10, 10, 10, 10, 10, 10, 10
Mean ± SD	**10 ± 20.4**	**10 ± 2.4**
p (significantly different from zero)		
	ns	**< 0.000**

2.9 Conclusions and examples

1. For ethicists crossover/self-controlled designs frequently are less a problem than
parallelgroup designs.
2. If the number of tests in a trial is a more important determinant of costs than the time
required for the trial, selfcontrolled/crossover trials are more cost effective.

3. If we have a small group of test subjects for a trial, f.e., 10 to 20, a parallelgroup study does not make sense because of lack of statistical power. A selfcontrolled/crossover design would, however, be no problem.

4. A trial dependent on subjective variables, f.e., clinical symptoms should have a parallel-group design.

5. A trial of curative treatments should have a parallel-group design unless it is a phase 1-2 acute study.

6. Unstable diseases, influenced, f.e., by seasonal effects, should be studied by parallel-group designs, unless phase 1-2 acute studies are involved.

7. Studies comparing treatment modalities with a negative between-treatment correlation, should not have a crossover/self-controlled design.

Example 1: an angina pectoris study, that studies nifedipine and nitroglycerin versus placebo should not be crossover because of a presumably negative correlation between nifedipine and nitroglycerin, since nitroglycerin is supposed to be more effective for angina with increased preload, while nifedipine is so in the case of Prinz-metall angina. Because of the possibly life-threatening aspect of the condition, it would seem unethical to have a parallel-group on placebo in this trial. The solution is a treatment comparison between nitroglycerin and nifedipine using a parallel-group design preferably without a placebo-arm in the study. To enhance power the sample size may have to be increased.

Example 2: the investigators of the effect of slow release nitroglycerin tablets twice vs once daily on angina pectoris do not feature a parallel-group design because they have few patients and think that between-subject variability of symptoms would be fatal to their efforts. However, angina pectoris is essentially a pain syndrome that is estimated by subjective variables. So, a crossover seems not appropriate either. The solution would be a crossover with objective variables, f.e., numbers of additional sublingual nitroglycerin and mm's ST-depression on the electrocardiogram.

Acknowledgement

The author is indebted to the editor and publisher of the American Journal of Therapeutics for granting permission to use part of a paper previously published in the journal (1994; 1: 327-32).

References

1. Moser LE. Statistical concepts fundamental to investigators. N Engl J Med 1985; 312: 890-7.
2. Sitthi-Amorn C, Poshyachinda V. Bias. Lancet 1993; 342 (II): 286-8.
3. Griso JA. Making comparisons. Lancet 1993; 324 (II): 157-60.
4. Cleophas TJ, Bailar JC. Statistical concepts fundamental to investigations [letter]. N Engl J Med 1985; 313: 1026.
5. Harrison DG. Clinical testing of beta-adrenergic blockade in angina pectoris, in Morselli P.O., et al. (ed.): Laboratoires d'Etudes et de Recherches Synthelabo. Vol 1, New York, Raven Press 1983; 243-50.

6. Brown BW. The crossover experiment for clinical trials. Biometrics 1980; 36: 69-79.
7. Cleophas TJ. Testing Crossover studies for carryover effects. Angiology 1989; 40: 287-93.
8. Van Lier HJ, Cleophas TJ. The crossover design in cardiovascular research, Abstract Book, Annual Meeting. International College of Angiology, Montreux, Switzerland, ed. by the International College of Angiology, Roslyn. N.Y., 1987; p 41.
9. Willan AR, Pater JL. Carryover and the two-period clinical trial. Biometrics 1986; 42: 593-9.
10.Hills M, Armitage P. The two-period crossover trial. Br J Clin Pharmacol 1979; 8: 7-20.
11.Barker M, Hew RJ, Huitson A, Poloniecki J. The two period crossover trial. Bias 1982; 9: 67-112.
12.Cleophas TJ. Underestimation of treatment effect in crossover trials. Angiology 1990; 41: 855-64.
13.Cleophas TJ. Crossover studies: a modified analysis with more power. Clin Pharmacol Ther 1993; 53: 515-20.
14.Cleophas TJ. A simple method for the estimation of interaction bias in crossover studies. J Clin Pharmacol 1990; 30: 1036-40.
15.Cleophas TJ. The performance of the two-stage analysis of two-period crossover trials [letter]. Stat Med 1991; 10: 489-95.
16.Cleophas TJ, Niemeyer MG. Carryover effects in cardiovascular crossover studies: the standard and the clinical analysis. Angiology 1993; 44: 271-9.
17.Cleophas TJ. Interaction biases in two-period crossover studies: a modified analysis to test with more sensitivity. Biom J 1993; 35: 181-91.
18.Pocock SJ, Hughes MD, Lee RJ. Statistical problems in the reporting of clinical trials. N Engl J of Med 1987; 317: 426-32.
19.Packer M. Combined beta-adrenergic and calcium entry blockade in angina pectoris. N Engl J Med 1989; 320: 709-18.
20.Fleiss JL. A critique of recent research on the two-treatment crossover design. Controll Clin Trials 1989; 10: 237-44.
21.Grieve AP. A bayesian analysis of the two-period crossover design for clinical trials. Biometrics 1985; 41: 979-90.
22.Freeman PR. The performance of the two-stage analysis of two-treatment, two-period crossover trials. Stat Med 1989; 8: 1421-32.
23.Jones B, Kennard MG. Design and Analysis of Crossover Trials. New York: Routledge, Chapman & Hall, 1989.
24.Prescott RJ. The comparison of success rates in crossover trials in the presence of an order effect. Appl Stat 30: 9-15, 1981.
25.Cornfield J, O'Neill RT. Minutes of the food and drug administation, biostatistics and epidemiology Advisory Committee meeting, June 23, 1976.
26.Strathers AD, Dollery CT. Therapeutic approaches. In "Handbook of Hypertension". Doyle AE, ed., Elsevier, 1984, Amsterdam, 2-3.

CHAPTER 3

LACK OF REAL SCIENCE
OF SYMTOM-BASED CARE

Objective. The management of chronic benign diseases although the mainstay of many practices, has not been the focus of education of physicians. The resulting dissonance causes much dissatisfaction on the part of both providers and consumers of health care. We hypothesized that lack of real science in this area is an important element of this dissonance.

Data sources. In search for data in the field of symptom-based care we scanned important textbooks, published papers, and the opinions of faculty program officers of medical schools.

Study Selection. As criteria we used common symptoms of patients with chronic benign diseases as estimated by the presidents of the 42 Patient Protection Groups in the Netherlands.

Data Extraction. Data were extracted independently of the investigators by the librarians of our institution.

Data Synthesis: Textbooks and review articles provide little information on the management of symptom-based care. This is associated with a lack of clinical trials on this subject on the one hand and negative feelings about its relevance on the part of the universities on the other hand.

Conclusions. As both prosperity and mean age rise, the profession is becoming increasingly involved in the problems of patients with chronic benign diseases. Currently no real science in this field is available.

3.1   Introduction

Symptom-based management of chronic benign diseases although the mainstay of many practices has not been the focus of the education of most physicians. Skills and knowledge in this area are mainly learned in everyday practice and not in the context of a medical school or residency curriculum. The resulting dissonance causes much dissatisfaction on the part of both providers and consumers of health care. In the Netherlands 1 in 5 citizens (20%) is currently holding a membership of one of the 42 Patient Protection Groups unified in the state-aided "Working Party for Patients with Chronic Benign Diseases (WOCZ)" (Table I). The magnitude of this largest grouping of patients in the nation is indicative of such dissatisfaction on the part of the consumers. On the part of the providers the widely held prejudice [1] that chronic complaints are generally unaccessible to therapy is another expression of such dissatisfaction.

Universities teach that etiology is based on causal thinking. So is our concept of a disease. However, mankind is currently becoming increasingly involved in the problems of patients with chronic benign diseases. People do not usually die of these, nor do they recover. Apparently, the issues are essentially different here. There is generally little point in looking for causalities or treatments that cure. Priority, at least to patients, is that their symptoms and complaints are appropriately taken care of. This is, however, something that many professionals are not very good at, maybe because they haven't been sufficiently trained to that end. In addition, not too long ago symptom-based care was denigrated by the profession as unscientific and unprofessional and more appropriate in the realm of nursing. So far,there is no gold standard for physicians' performance of symptom-based care against which it can be judged. Obviously, we are dealing with an underdeveloped aspect of our discipline. In the current paper we hypothesize that lack of scientific evidence of symptom-based therapies is an important element of this dissonance.

Table I. 2.4 Million Dutch Citizens (17% of the whole nation) hold a membership of one of the patient protection groups unified in the state-aided "working Party for Patients with Chronic Benign Diseases (WOCZ)"

1. Addison's, Cushing's disease	22. Lupus erythematodes
2. Alzheimer's disease	23. Lymphedema
3. Bulimia	24. Meniere's syndrome
4. Celiac disease	25. Migraine
5. Cerebrovascular disease	26. Multiple sclerosis
6. Chronic dermatologic diseases	27. Muscle diseases
7. Chronic fatigue syndrome	28. Organic psychosyndrome
8. Chronic hepatitis	29. Osteogenesis imperfecta
9. Chronic obstructive pulmonary disease	30. Osteoporosis
10. Chronic pain	31. Parenteral feeding
11. Crohn, colitis	32. Parkinson's disease
12. Cystic fibrosis	33. Posttraumatic dystrophia
13. Diabetes	34. Psoriasis
14. Epilepsy	35. Pulmonary asthma
15. Fibromyalgia	36. Renal disease
16. Friedrich Wegener disease	37. Rheumatoid arthritis
17. Heart disease	38. Sarcoidosis
18. Heart transplants	39. Sjogren's syndrome
19. HIV	40. Thyroid diseases
20. Ileo- and Colostomy	41. Vascular diseases
21. Incontinence	42. Whiplash

3.2   Methods

In order to estimate the amount of scientific knowledge available we scanned the following material:

1. Material on the issue of symptom-based care independent of disease as available in important textbooks.
2. Published papers of clinical trials on the subject as available in the years 1990-1995 of MEDLINE database [5].
3. Review articles on the subject as available in the 1990-1995 volumes of two important general journals: JAMA and the NEJM.
4. Faculty programs of the 8 medical schools in the Netherlands for their assessment of symptom-based care in their curricula.

3.3   Study selection and data extraction

Presidents of the 42 Patient Protection Groups in the Netherlands were questioned to provide without our assistance a listing of the most common symptoms and complaints of patients with chronic benign diseases. When searching Textbooks and publications in JAMA and the NEJM we used these symptoms and complaints as searchterms. When searching MEDLINE data we did so in combination with the following keywords: clinical trial (or study), controlled trial, randomized trial, experimental trial, crossover trial, and parallel trial. Data were extracted independently of the investigators by the librarians of our institution.

3.4   Data synthesis

Textbooks (Table II)
Harrison's Principles of Internal Medicine [3] offers a whole 266 of its 2204 pages to "Cardinal Symptoms of Disease". This part of the book focuses on symptoms important to patients with chronic benign diseases. However, the point of therapy for such symptoms was usually either not raised or answered rather superficially by a formulation such as: therapy depends on the correction of the underlying cause. In Cecil's Textbook of Medicine [4] (2380 pages) a section on symptoms independent of disease is missing. Maybe, it is therefore that items such as indigestion, and malaise could not be found at all. The other items were addressed at different places in the text in a very much similar way.

Published papers (Table III)
The librarians of our institution were questioned to go through the years 1990-1995 of MEDLINE database[5]. Table III shows that virtually no controlled randomized trials have been published on the assessment or treatment of the items considered by the presidents of the Patient Protection Groups. In the same period of time MEDLINE Database encountered approximately 48,000 controlled randomized trials on hypertension. So,our database system was not a small one.

Table II. Information about symtom-based therapies for patients with chronic benign diseases as offered by textbooks

Cecil's Textbook of Medicine	Harrison's Principles of Internal Medicine
l. Anemia: it is the most frequent and significant world-wide health problem and remains a cardinal indicator of disease which requires careful evaluation	effective therapy is predicated upon a thorough diagnostic evaluation
2. Anorexia: the depression of appetite in gastrointestinal disease is not well inderstood	the mechanism is poorly understood
3. Chronic fatigue: if not explained by a careful search for causes, it often has a psychogenic basis	- therapy not mentioned -
4. Chronic pain: is best treated by treating underlying disorders	patients with chronic pain present special problems in management
5. Constipation: when treatable diseases are excluded it is important to educate the patient	patients should be shifted away from the quixotic search for perfect stool resulting from an inordinate expectation of regularity
6. Dizziness: best treatment is successful treatment of underlying disease	-therapy not mentioned -
7. Dysphagia: defined as hypothalamic eating disorder	dependent upon cause
8. Fatigue: a prominant symptom of chronic disorders and a major underlying challenge for the physician	expression of underlying depression
9. Gait disorder: -item not addressed-	-item not addressed-
l0. Gustatory loss: no specific treatment, attention to underlying illness	therapy remains limited
ll. Headache: the best treatment is prevention *i.e.* avoiding of precipitating factors	the most important steps in the treatment are measures which uncover the underlying disease or disturbance
12. Impotence: medical therapy offers little more than placebo effect and may actually delay identification of underlying disorders that have been overlooked	-therapy not mentioned-
13. Incontinence: -item not addressed-	-item not addressed -
14. Indigestion: -therapy not mentioned-	-therapy not mentioned-
15. Irritability, Depression, and related psychological problems: -not addressed-	-not addressed-
16. Malaise: -therapy not mentioned-	-therapy not mentioned-
17. Nausea: -therapy not mentioned	depends on correction of underlying cause

Table II (continued). Information about symtom-based therapies for patients with chronic benign diseases as offered by textbooks

Cecil's Textbook of Medicine	Harrison's Principles of Internal Medicine
18. Pruritus: usually there are no dermatologic findings. To date no single causative factor has been identified	it is often the expression of an underlying systemic disease
19. Reduced concentration and memory: -not addressed-	-not addressed-
20. Reduced physical condition: -not addressed -	-not addressed-
21. Refractory edema: no therapy, only differential diagnoses	-therapy not mentioned-
22. Shortness of breath: there is no category of medications for relief independent of cause	in most patients the dyspnea is relieved after disease of heart of heart or lungs are treated
23. Sensory loss: -therapy not mentioned	-therapy not mentioned-
24. Sleep disruption: conservative (=no) treatment is not likely to dangerous	the first principle is the recognition that the severity reported is often exaggerated
25. Weight loss: gastric surgery, malabsorption syndromes are major cause	is predominantly diagnostic problem

Review Articles in General Journals (Table IV)
In search for review articles on symptoms important to patients with chronic diseases we scanned the 1990-1995 volumes of JAMA and the NEJM. JAMA published only 51 reviews and none of them emphasized therapeutic considerations. We should add that otherwise the subject of chronic benign diseases was addressed quite frequently in JAMA, particularly in the context of governmental issues, insurance matters, general health care, epidemiology and preventive medicine. The NEJM published 303 review articles mainly on the issue of molecular medicine and pathophysiology. Only 7 of these articles addressed such symptoms. The emphasis in these articles was on diagnostic work-up rather than therapy.

Faculty program offices (Table V)
We contacted by telephone faculty officers of the 8 medical schools in the Netherlands. Table V gives an overview of the answers to the questions we addressed. None of the medical schools offer any course on symtom-based care at this time. Two schools were opposed to the idea to develop one. These two schools expressed that they considered training in differential diagnosis far more important and stressed that symptomatic medicine might be counter-productive to diagnosis making, and eventually lead to less knowledgeable physicians. This, then, could very well result in harm being done to certain categories of patients.

Table III. Randomized controlled trials 1991-1995*. Few data in the field of symtom-based care of patients with chronic benign diseases are offered by scientific papers as compared to hypertension data.

Number of controlled randomized trials 1990-1995*	
1. Anemia	4
2. Anorexia	3
3. Chronic fatigue	-
4. Chronic pain	3
5. Constipation	3
6. Dizziness	-
7. Dysphagia	-
8. Fatigue	-
9. Gait disorder	-
10. Gustatory loss	-
11. Headache	-
12. Impotence	5
13. Incontinence	-
14. Indigestion	-
15. Irritability	-
16. Malaise	-
17. Nausea	-
18. Pruritus	13
19. Reduced memory	-
20. Reduced physical condition	-
21. Refractory edema	-
22. Shortness of breath	-
23. Sensory loss	-
24. Sleep disruption	-
25. Weight loss	10
Hypertension +ACE inhibitors	3,681
Hypertension +calcium antagonists	6,083
Hypertension	47,792

* Estimation based on MEDLINE Database [5].

3.5   Discussion

Textbook and general journals provide little information on symptom-based care independent of disease. Specialist journals may be more willing than general journals to publish experts' views on this topic. For example, the European Journal of Gastroen-terology recently published a review of the management of chronic diarrhea, and unlike the NEJM and JAMA (Table III) came to the conclusion that anti-diarrhea drugs have an extremely valuable part in the management [6]. In recent years specialist journals have also been engaged in publishing consensus views when data were inadequate.

Table IV. Information about symptom-based therapies for patients with chronic diseases as offered by review articles in JAMA and NEJM 1990-1995.

JAMA	
Review articles	n=51
Reviews on the items of Table 2	n=0

JAMA published 5 articles in the category Reviews. the Remaining 46 papers were considered by us because there was mentioning of review of literature either in "summary", "title" or "conclusions". None of the articles considered symptom-based therapies for patients with chronic diseases specifically.

NEJM	
Review articles	n=303
Reviews on the items of Table 2	n=7

Gait disorders 1990; 322: 1441	The best outcome is achieved when a specific condition is identified, a treatable disorder turns up roughly one of four cases; even so, patients are served well by a careful diagnostic procedure.
Sleep disorder 1990; 232: 520	Physicians need to consider a complex array of potential causes, the use of hypnotic drugs are clearly contraindicated.
Diarrhea 1190; 323: 891	None of the drug studied to date are of sufficient benefit and safety to justify their use in diarrhea. Referenced by a single paper from JAMA (1976; 236: 844: "Antidiarrhea Agents").
Incontinence 1992; 326: 1002	Careful diagnostic work-up is required.
Constipation and irritable bowel 1193; 329:1940	They represent a heterogeneous group of disorders. Efforts to investigate pathophysiologic mechanisms will lead to more effective therapy.
Diarrhea 1995; 332: 725	As our understanding improves, more patients will be found to have an organic rather than functional disorder.
Shortness of breath 1995; 333: 1547	The capacity to alleviate symptoms depends on our ability to define the mechanisms.

Such an approach generally identifies even more clearly that further research in this area is needed. For example, a COPD-consensus [7] stated that the progression of chronic obstructive pulmonary diseases (COPD) cannot be stopped and that a basis for symptom-based care in the form of controlled studies is missing. Similarly, a cardiac failure consensus [8] concluded that there is no cure other than transplantation, and that in the meantime symptomatic treatment must be based on current information until trials have provided unequivocal evidence.

The current report is based on the European experience. In the United States the management of chronic diseases is taking on increasing importance in the education of both medical students and house-staff, as outpatient training gains equal status with inpatient training. At the same time, the Cochrane collaboration and evidence-based medicine movement are active in telling educators to shift balance away from expert opinion toward evidence, ie randomized clinical trials [9]. In so doing, however, this movement unintentionally participates in the current publication bias of publishing mainly glamorous research and not taking up more common topics such as symptom-based care of chronic diseases.

For decisions made in everyday clinical practice where results of randomized clinical trials are missing, an alternative to expert opinions may be a registry of cases.

Information could be gathered on all patients who present to hospitals within a defined area. This process could be facilitated with preformatted forms outlining the data we wish to collect. Within a short time it might be possible to obtain answers to so far unanswered questions. As a matter of fact, this procedure has been used to establish that octreotide was effective for the treatment of chronic diarrhea associated with short bowel syndrome [14], antineoplastic drugs [15], and diabetic neuropathy [16], but not acute diarrhea [17].

Palliative care is considered to be different from symptom-based management in that the former is supposed to deal with issues in the management of terminally ill and the latter is related to a variety of ailments suffered by the person [14]. The hospice literature usually embraces the former and no literature by and large has taken up the latter. Also, quality of life studies are considered to be different [15,16]. Although they focus on symptoms and adverse effects,they do so in the context of treatments given for indications other than the relief of such symptoms, for example, the remission of cancer, or the reduction of blood pressure.

Table V. Answers of the Faculty Program Officers of the 8 Medical Schools in the Netherlands to Questions Addressing the Assessment of Symptom-based Therapies in their Curriculum.

	Answer is yes (n=8)	
1. Courses on symtom-based therapies currently given	0	0%
2. In favor of the idea to start such courses	0	0%
3. Current courses on general symptoms of disease emphasizing differential diagnosis rather than treatment regimens	3	38%
4. In favor of shifting such emphasis towards symptom based care	0	0%
5. Definitely opposed to this very idea	2	25%

The management of chronic diseases should, of course, not be equated with symptom-based care, since other important aspects of management such as prevention of complications and treatment of the underlying disorders would be precluded. Second, it would be folly to establish symptom-based practices without consideration to the underlying chronic diseases. The management of a patient with shortness of breath, for example, would depend largely on whether the patient had one or more of the following disorders: COPD, congestive heart failure, coronary artery disease with angina, chronic anemia, or poor endurance from deconditioning. Third, patients with chronic benign diseases have other priorities that should be taken into account as well, ie, social and financial problems, side effects from chronic treatments given, comorbidity such as enhanced susceptibility to thrombo-embolic complications, respiratory and gastro-intestinal morbidity. Even so, many patients with various types of chronic diseases suffer from recurrent symptoms that persist even if their underlying condition has been carefully taken care of and for which the medical community has little treatment to offer. COPD is the third most common cause of incapacity in Europe [7]. Chronic cardiac failure ranks as second most common cardiac cause of hospitalization in elderly, and its incidence is steeply rising [8]. In such diagnosis groups symptoms of, for example, shortness of breath and fatigue usually persist even if underlying conditions have been appropriately taken care of. Whether such symptoms can be alleviated by physiotherapy, psychological reinforcement or respiratory stimulants would be the subject of a suitable trial for symptom-based care.

The fact that we have no real science of symptom-based care independent of disease should not be taken to mean that there has been no philosophical attention to this area [17]. The whole area of phenomenology and medicine is in part based on these considerations [18]. There is enough substance here for faculties to start building a body of science upon. It is time for faculties to start doing so. There is one more reason for doing so. Obviously, there is a growing market for this very kind of care (Table I).

Acknowledgement

The author is indebted to the editor and publisher of Clinical Research And Regulatory Affairs for granting permission to use parts of a paper previously published in the journal (1996; 13: 167-79).

References

1. Buchanan A, Bhugra B. Attitude of the medical profession to the treatment of chronic pain. Acta Psych Scand 1992; 85: 1- 5.
2. Cleophas TJM. Clinical trials in chronic diseases: new endpoints. Clin Research & Reg Affairs 1995; 12:273-82.
3. Wilson JD, Braunwald E, Isselbacher KJ, eds Harrison's Principles of Internal Medicine, McGraw-Hill Inc, NY, 1991 (12th edition).
4. Wijngaarden JB, Smith L II, eds Cecil's Textbook of Medicine, Saunders, Philadelphia, 1992 (19th edition).
5. Medline Database, U.S. National Library of Medicine, Washington DC, 1995.
6. Farthing MJG. Chronic diarrhea: current concepts on mechanisms and management. Eur J Gastroenterol 1996; 8: 157-69.
7. Siatakas NM, Vermeire P, Prive NB, for the European Respiratory Society. Optimal assessment and management of chronic obstructive pulmonary disease. Eur Resp J 1995; 8: 1398-420.
8. Burkart F, Erdman E, Hanrath P, for the German Society for Cardiovascular Research. Consensus Conference "Therapy of chronic heart insufficiency". Zeitschr Kardiol 1993; 82: 200-10.

9. Evidence-based Medicine Working Group. A new approach to teaching the practice of medicine. JAMA 1992; 268: 2420-5.

10. Nightingale JMD, Lennard-Jones JE, Walker EB, Farthing MJG. Jejunal reflux in short bowel syndrome. Lancet 1990; 336: 765-8.

11. Fetrelli NJ. Continous high-dose infusion of octreotide acetate for treatment of chemotherapy - induced diarrhea in patients with colorectal cancer. Cancer 1993; 72: 177-82.

12. Mourad FH, Gorard D, Thillainayagram AV, Colin-Jones D. Effective treatment of diabetic diarrhea with octreotide. Gut 1992; 33: 1578-80.

13. Burrough AK, McCormick PA. Somatostatin and octreotide in gastroenterology. Aliment Pharmacol Ther 1991; 5: 331-41.

14. Anonymous. The inhumanity and humanity of medicine. Dying for palliative care. BMJ 1994; 309: 1696-9.

15. Gill TM,Feinstein AR. A critical appraisal of the quality of life measurements. JAMA 1994; 272: 619-26.

16. Wilson JB,Cleary PD. Linking clinical variables with health-related quality of life. JAMA 1995; 273: 59-65.

17. Kant I. Kritik der Urteilskraft. DrMax Janecke, Verlagsbuchhandlung, Leipzig, 1920.

18. McManus IC. Humanity and the medical humanities. Lancet 1995; 346: 1143-5.

CHAPTER 4

CARRYOVER EFFECTS IN CLINICAL RESEARCH

If the effect of a treatment carries on after the treatment is withdrawn then the response to a second treatment may well be due in part to the previous treatment. This, so called, carryover effect may bias any clinical trial in which subjects are tested more than once. Crossover studies can be routinely checked for this bias. In other study designs, however, common sense and alertness for unusual patterns in the data are the only defenses against it.

The amount of carryover bias in clinical trials can be somewhat minimized by the following measures. Dose response studies, dose titration studies, and open evaluation studies should require a sufficient washout period between the administrations of the drugs. Studies using duplicate standard deviations for the estimation of intraindividual reproducibility of a test, should routinely include a statistical test for differences between the duplicate data. Self-controlled studies should not be used otherwise than as an initial orientation on a new treatment. Parallel studies should routinely be stratified for symmetry of previous treatments. Studies with subjective variables are frequently influenced by psychological carryover effects and should, therefore, be validated together with objective variables whenever possible. In spite of these measures many cases of carryover effect remain unpreventable.

4.1   Introduction

If the effect of one treatment carries on after the treatment is withdrawn then the response to a second treatment may well be due in part to the previous treatment. This is the so called carryo effect. It is usually thought of as a physical carryover effect of a compound in the blood stream. However, another real possibility is that of psychological carryover. The term was first used in conjunction with crossover trials [1-4], where each patient serves as his own control. Procedures have been developed to test for carryover effect in such studies [5-12]. From them one may conclude that carryover effect may have a large impact on the final results and may largely invalidate these studies. The FDA [13] and some statisticians [1,14-17] even discouraged the use of crossovers because of this potential bias. Using the standard phase 1-4 classification of clinical trials [11,18,19] (Table I), I demonstrate that carryover effect may not only bias crossovers, but also any other type of clinical trial in which subjects are tested more than once.

Table I.   Phase 1-4 Classification of clinical trials

		characteristics	popular study designs
Phase	1-2	. normal volunteers . pharmacokinetics, biologic effects dose titration	. dose response studies . dose titration studies . studies with duplicate standard deviations
Phase	2-3	. small groups of patients . therapeutic efficacy, and safety	. open evaluation studies . crossover studies . self-controlled studies
Phase	3-4	. large groups of patients . longterm effects, quality of life assessment, postmarketing surveillance	. parallel-group studies . studies with subjective variables

4.2   Dose Response and Dose Titration Studies

A dose-effect relationship is commonly derived from the effect after a series of incremental doses of a drug. A dose response study estimates this effect by use of mean scores. A dose titration study does so by % responders. In the classical receptor theory it is assumed that the drug effect is proportional to the fraction of receptors occupied by the drug and that maximal effect occurs when all receptors are occupied. The Michaelis Menten equation explains the shape of the dose response and dose titration curves.

$$\text{Effect} = \frac{\text{Maximal Effect x Dose}}{\text{Constant + Dose}}$$

This equation describes a simple hyperbola with the maximal effect approached asymptotically. In order to display a wide range of drugconcentrations more easily, log dose is frequently plotted instead of dose. Thus, the result is the familiar sigmoidal log dose - effect curve (Figure 1). Anomalous relationships may result from different causes, f.e., a maximal response from less than maximal receptor occupancy (spare receptors), from a threshold phenomenon or from the presence of compatitive agents in the blood. Anomalous curves, especially very steep ones (Figure 1), may be caused by carryover effect because of the following. In dose response studies the subjects are generally tested several times. The second experiment usually takes place after 4 plasma halftimes of the drug that is tested. Figure 2 shows that even after 4 halftimes the plasma level is not yet zero and that after a two-fold dosage the plasma level at 4 halftimes is equally two-fold. In addition, a significant receptor occupancy may last longer than 4 plasma halftimes. These effects, although assumed by statisticians [20] are not routinely taken into account by investigators. Their result would be an overestimation of treatment effect and recommendation of erroneously low doses in follow-up studies, giving rise to insufficient results. To test these assumptions we performed a dose response study of different doses the vasodilator phenoxybenzamine on finger temperature after standard finger cooling [21] in patients with Raynaud's disease (Figure 3). With 14 plasma halftime intervals between the subsequent doses the mean dose response relationship was significantly more flat (dotted curve). An interval of 4 plasma halftimes was apparently not sufficient to prevent a significant carryover effect (solid curve).

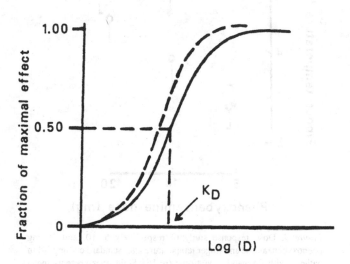

Figure 1. Dose (D) response curves with (—) and without (-) carryover effect due to accumulation of residual drug.

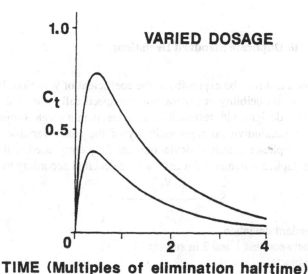

Figure 2. Patterns to illustrate the influence of a two-fold difference in dosage. Ct = concentration of drug in plasma(mg/l)at time t.

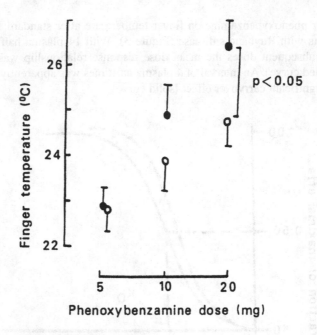

Figure 3. Dose response study of respectively 5, 10, and 20 mg phenoxybenzamine and finger temperature after standard cooling [4] in patients with Raynaud's syndrome (n=16). Solid lines presents mean results ± SD's of tests performed with 4 plasma halftime intervals between the tests, dotted line with 14 plasma halftimes.

4.3   Studies with Duplicate Standard Deviations

Reproducibility of a test may be expressed as the coefficient of variation. However, this method measures reproducibility in general and not specifically intra-individual reproducibility. For study designs with repeated measurements in a single subject an a priori assessment of the intraindividual reproducibility of the main variables is required. For that purpose duplicate standard deviations are frequently used. All subjects are tested twice. The duplicate standard deviations are calculated according to

$$S = \frac{V_i^{\,2}}{2n}$$

S = duplicate standard deviation
V_i = difference between test 1 and 2 in subject i
n = number of subjects

Table II gives a hypothesized example of such a procedure. In the left column there is a significant difference between test 1 and 2. In the right there is not. Still both columns have the same duplicate standard deviations. The significant difference between test 1 and 2 in the left column is probably due to carryover effect provided that the investigators kept the study circumstances of test series 1 and 2 at a constant level. From the example it can be seen that the duplicate standard deviations cannot differentiate between random effects and carryover bias. We recommend, therefore, always to combine duplicate standard deviations calculations with a statistical test for differences between the duplicates. If a significant difference is detected, the use of duplicate standard deviations has little value because it does not represent intra-individual reproducibility, but mainly carryover bias.

Table II. Two hypothesized studies with duplicate standard deviations

Subject (n=10)	Results		Subject (n=10)	Results	
	Test 1	Test 2		Test 1	Test 2
1	10	11	1	10	9
2	10	11	2	10	11
3	10	11	3	10	9
4	10	11	4	10	11
5	10	11	5	10	9
6	10	11	6	10	11
.	.	.	.	.	.
.	.	.	.	.	.
.	.	.	.	.	.
	$p < 0.000$			N.S.	
	Duplicate Standard			Duplicate Standard	
	Deviation $1/2 \sqrt{2}$			Deviation $1/2 \sqrt{2}$	

4.4 Open Evaluation Studies

Carryover effects may also occur when different compounds are administered after each other. Even completely new and unexpected effects may result from interactions between the different compounds that are present in the blood stream together. For example, we studied the effects of different adrenergic receptor agonists and antagonists on the blood pressure of normotensive subjects. Phenoxybenzamine hardly influenced the blood pressure, whereas epinephrine caused a substantial rise in blood pressure (Figure 4). However, when epinephrine was given after phenoxybenzamine, the pressor effect turned into a depressor. This effect was explained by a carryover effect of phenoxybenzamine, blocking the vasoconstrictive alpha-receptors and giving rise to a beta-vasodilator

effect of epinephrine. Similarly an enhanced pressor effect of epinephrine can be observed
after pretreatment with propranolol which is a compound that otherwise decreased
the blood pressure. Such interactions are common in all day clinical practice where sick
subjects are given a number of drugs until their equilibrium is restored. It is, of course,
impossible to evaluate the effects of the separate compounds in these situations. It is,
however, essential to do so in open evaluation studies of new pharmacological compounds.
In such studies a number of newly developed compounds is given shortly after each
other to a single subject or a small group of subjects. This is done for the purpose of
a fast selection of a few compounds for further study. Because of economical reasons
such studies are frequently uncontrolled. At least, they should have appropriate washout
periods between two tests, just like dose response and dose titration studies require.
Otherwise results are likely to be biased by carryover effects.

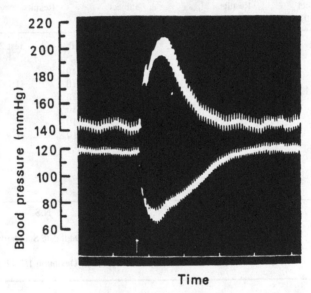

Figure 4. Response of blood pressure to epinephrine with and without
prior administration of phenoxybenzamine
(lower and upper record respectively).

4.5   Crossover Studies

Table III shows the basic design of a crossover study. Group A receives the test compound in the first period followed by placebo or standard therapy. Group B receives
the two treatments in the reverse order. In the analysis the data of the test compound
periods are taken together and compared with the data of the placebo or standard therapy
periods (a + d versus c + b). Physical carryover effect occurs when a treatment is used to

cure rather than alleviate. Suppose the test compound is an antibiotic (Table IV). After period 1, 100% of the patients in group A and 0% of the patients in group B are cured. After the next period, finally all patients are cured. In the analysis the difference between antibiotic and placebo in group A is zero; in group B it is 100% - mean value 50% improvement. Obviously a crossover design should never be used when a treatment cures a disease. However, also with symptomatic therapies, small curative effects can occur, f.e., wound healing by vasodilators. This is illustrated by a study of Kahan [22] (Table V). Efficacy of a vasodilator is assessed in patients with Raynaud's syndrome. Group A has the placebo after the vasodilator. The frequency of Raynaud attacks is only 25 attacks per week. Group B has the placebo first. The score is not less than 34.3 attacks which is significantly different from 25 (p < 0.05). Analyzing the data according to the crossover design we find an improvement in group A of -1 attack, and in group B of -11,2 attacks, mean improvement -6.1 attacks. But when we just forget period 2 and compare the data of the first period, the improvement is -10.3 attacks. So, the crossover gives a more than 40% underestimation compared with the first period. This is probably largely due to a physical carryover effect in group A. The beneficial vasodilator effect in this group seems to carry on after the compound has been withdrawn and replaced by placebo.

Table III. Study designs

	Crossover Study				
	Period 1			Period 2	
	Treatment	Mean Efficacy		Treatment	Mean Efficacy
Group A	New Therapy	a		Standard Therapy*	c
Group B	Standard Therapy	b		New Therapy	d
	Self-controlled Study				
	Period 1			Period 2	
	Treatment	Mean Efficacy		Treatment	Mean Efficacy
Single Group	Standard Therapy	a		New Therapy	b
	Parallel-group Study				
	Single period				
	Treatment	Mean Efficacy			
Group A	New Therapy	a			
Group B	Standard Therapy	b			

* Instead of standard therapy, placebo is frequently used.

Table IV. Model of crossover study with antibiotic or placebo

	Period 1		Period 2	
	Treatment	Mean Efficacy*	Treatment	Mean Efficacy
Group A	Antibiotic	100%	Placebo	100%
Group B	Placebo	0%	Antibiotic	100%

* Percentage of cured patients

Table V. Efficacy of vasodilator or placebo in a crossover study in patients with Raynaud's syndrome [22]

	Period 1		Period 2	
	Treatment	Mean Efficacy*	Treatment	Mean Efficacy
Group A (n=10)	Vasodilator	24.0 ± 11.0	Placebo	25.0 ± 10.8
Group B (n=10)	Placebo	34.3 ± 14.9	Vasodilator	23.1 ± 19.1

* Mean frequency of Raynaud attacks/week S.D.

4.6   Self-controlled Studies

These are studies, where a single group of patients is given a standard treatment and a new treatment after each other (Table III). Similarly to crossovers a carryover effect from period 1 into period 2 is possible. However, an additional problem is, that, since a control group is missing here, data cannot be tested for it. The next problem is, that self-controlled studies are more often used at early points in the development of new treatments [23], so that we have few clinical arguments against carryover effect. An additional weakness of such studies is the general use of large numbers of variables [23] enhancing the chance of a type II error of finding a difference where there is none and of confounding of dependent and independent variables because multivariate analysis is rarely applied. This, all in all, means that self-controlled trials should not be used otherwise than as an initial orientation on a new treatment. One exception is the situation where a trial is designed in order to detect carryover effect. F.e., Packer *et al.* [24] used a self-controlled study to investigate the clinical reaction of patients with heart failure to acute withdrawal of nitroprussid. The self-controlled design seems ideal for the establishment of this rebound phenomenon, which can be considered as a special form of carryover effect [24].

4.7   Parallel-Group Studies

In parallel-group studies two groups of patients receive a different treatment throughout the trial (Table III). Because there is no change-over of therapy during the trial, carry-over effects within the trial are excluded. However, carryover effects from treatments prior to the trial are not and may bias parallel studies to a greater extent than they do crossovers. The point is that the between-group comparison of parallel studies is much more dependent on symmetry of the treatment groups than the within group comparison of crossovers. This can be illustrated by a parallel-group study of Graham on the effect of positive-pressure or sham ventilation on patients with pneumonia [25]. The treatment group was significantly better than the control group. Although three of the four co-variates were almost evenly split between the treatment groups, the fourth (prior anti-biotic treatment) was somewhat lopsided (Table VI). Because prior antibiotic therapy was likely to have a clinically large effect on outcome, the imbalance could easily have biased the results. We recommend that during randomization parallel groups should not only routinely be stratified for symmetry of covariates such as age, sex, duration of sickness but also for symmetry of previous treatments.

Table VI. Patients' characteristics in a two-group parallel study of positive-pressure ventilation treatment for pneumonia[25]

	Control Group	Treatment Group
Total no. of patients	27	27
No. of men	13	14
Age (years)	63	61
No. of smokers	16	17
No. who took antibiotics before admission	5	10

4.8   Studies with Subjective Variables

Another real possibility is that of psychological carryover. This can be illustrated by a simple crossover design (Table III). A less active agent is compared with an effective one and both treatments are judged by a subjective variable, f.e., improvement of complaints. In the first period with the effective agent most patients feel reduction in complaints. They approach the second with confidence. The other group experiences little improvement and gets a bad feeling about the trial. This influences its appraisal of the second period. Table VII gives an example: Group A received a new effective vasodilator before standard therapy and had a better score than Group B, 2.2 versus 1.8 points (new vasodilator Group A versus Group B, $p < 0.05$). The difference between the new and standard therapy in Group A was 2.2-1.2 = 1.0 point. In group B 1.8-1.2 = 0.6 point - mean value 0.8 point. But when we just forget about period 2 and compare the data of the first period, the improvement is 2.2-1.2 = 1.0 point. So this crossover gives underestimation, some 20%. This is probably due to a psychological carryover effect in Group B. The patients in this group are disappointed and this impairs their appraisal of the second period. This example deals with psychological carryover effect in a crossover design. The test subject's attitude to a study is, however, a variable hard to control in any study design. For example, most of the placebo-controlled parallel studies will have run in periods either with placebo or with an active agent. This may cause similarly either a negative or a positive psychological carryover effect from the very start. Moreover, the subjects of the placebo arm of the study may lose their motivation during the trial giving rise to underestimation of the final result of this arm rather than proper estimation of it. Also cohort or case-control studies using multiple questionnaires may suffer from this type of gradual demotivation bias that is hardly given any attention by the scientific community so far. Psychological carryover effects can of course be minimized by the use of objective variables (f.e., physical measurements like blood pressure, heart rate, temperature). Subjective variables are, however, frequently indispensible and may even be the only ones that count.

What is the good of a treatment if it does not make you feel better? A defense against the potential bias from psychological carryover effects is alertness at unusual patterns of answers. Unfortunately, there is generally no statistical method to test for it. Also, the value of subjective data should be validated together with objective variables and be interpreted with caution.

Table VII. Efficacy of two Vasodilators a crossover study in patients with Raynaud's syndrome[26]

	Period 1		Period 2	
	Treatment	Mean Efficacy*	Treatment	Mean Efficacy
Group A	New Vasodilator	2.2 ± 0.8	StandardVasodilator	1.2 ± 0.9
Group B	Standard Vasodilator	1.2 ± 0.8	New Vasodilator	1.8 ± 0.6

* Mean improvement of Raynaud complaints ± SD., judged by a 4-point clinical scale
(0 = no improvement; 4= complete relief).

4.9 Discussion

Carryover effect occurs when the response to a second treatment is in part due to the previous part of the study. It was first described in connection with crossover studies [1-4]. From previous statistical reports one may conclude that it may have a large impact on the final results and may largely invalidate these studies [3,4,14,16]. The present paper shows that substantial carryover bias may also occur in any other type of study where subjects are treated more than once, while there are virtually no methods to test for it. So, there is little one can do to address this bias in these situations. The following recommendations may be considered by investigators:

1. Crossover studies should routinely include a statistical test for carryover bias. Simple methods for this purpose are the Grizzle test [1] or the "look at the data method" [9,27].

2. In other study designs no test is available. So, clinical arguments and alertness for unexpected patterns in the data are the only defenses against it so far.

3. Dose response, dose titration, and open evaluation studies should require sufficient washout periods between the administrations of the drugs. Even 14 plasma halftimes may be required.

4. Studies using of duplicate standard deviations should always be combined with a statistical test for differences between the duplicate data. If a significant difference is detected, the use of duplicate standard deviations for the estimation of intra-individual reproducibility has little value.

5. Self-controlled studies, should not be used otherwise than as an initial orientation on a new treatment.

6. Parallel studies should routinely be stratified for symmetry of previous treatments.

7. Subjective variables are frequently exposed to psychological carryover effects. They should, therefore, be validated together with objective variables whenever possible. If not, they should be interpreted with caution.

8. Many cases of carryover bias seem unpreventable, we shall simply have to accept them.

Acknowledgement

Parts of this chapter have been previously published in the European Journal of Clinical Chemistry/Clinical Biochemistry (1993; 31: 803-09).

References

1. Grizzle JE. The two period change-over design and its use in clinical trials. Biometrics 1974; 30: 727-34.
2. Hills M, Armitage P. The two-period crossover trial. Br J Clin Pharmacol 1979; 8: 7-20.
3. Barker M, Hew RJ, Huitson A, Poloniecki J. The two period crossover trial. Bias 1982; 9: 67-112.
4. Cleophas TJ. Underestimation of treatment effect in crossover trials. Angiology 1990; 41: 855-64.
5. Brown BW. The crossover experiment for clinical trials. Biometrics 1980; 36: 69-79. 6. Cleophas TJ, Bailar JC. Statistical concept fundamental to investigations. N Engl J Med 1985; 313: 1026.
7. Cleophas TJ. Testing Crossover studies for carryover effects. Angiology 1989; 40: 287- 93.

8. Cleophas TJ. A simple method for the estimation of interaction bias in crossover studies. J Clin Pharmacol 1990; 30: 1036-40.

9 Cleophas TJ. The performance of the two- stage analysis of two-period crossover trials. Stat Med 1991; 10: 489-95.

10. Cleophas TJ. Interaction bias in crossover studies: a modified analysis to test with more sensitivity. Biometrical J 1993; 35: 181-91.

11. Kaitin KJ, Richard BW, Lasagna L. Trends in drug development: the 1985-86 new drug approvals. J Clin Pharmacol 1987; 27: 542-8.

12. Pocock SJ, Hughes MD, Lee RJ. Statistical problems in the reporting of clinical trials. N Engl J Med 1987; 317: 426-32.

13. Cornfield J, O'Neill RT. Minutes of the Food and Drug Administration. Biostatics and Epidemiology Advisory Committee meeting, June 23, 1976.

14. Fleiss JL. A critique of recent research on the two treatment crossover design. Controll Clin Trials 1989; 10: 237-44.

15. Freeman PR. The performance of the two-stage analysis of two-treatment, two-period crossover trials. Stat Med 1989; 8: 1421-32.

16. Grieve AP. A bayesian analysis of the two- period crossover design for clinical trials. Biometrics 1985; 41: 979-90.

17. Jones B, Kennard MG. Design and Analysis of Crossover Trials. Chapman and Hall, NY, 1989.

18. Nies AS. Principles of therapeutics. In: Goodman and Gilman's Pharmacological Basis of Therapeutics. ed. by Goodman A et al., Pergamon Press, NY, 1991, 62-83.

19. Young FE, Norris JA, Levitt JA, Nightingale SL. The FDA's new procedure for the use of investigational drugs in treatment. JAMA 1988; 250: 2267-70.

20. Sheiner LB, Hashimoto Y, Beal SL. A simulation study comparing designs for dose ranging. Stat Med 1991; 10: 303-23.

21. Cleophas TJ, Fennis JF, Van 't Laar A. Finger temperature after a finger cooling test. J Appl Physiol 1982; 52: 1167-71.

22. Kahan A, Amor B, Menkes CJ. Nicardipine in the treatment of Raynaud's phenomenon. Angiology 1987; 38: 333-7.

23. Louis TA, Lavori PW, Bailar JC, Polansky M. Crossover and self-controlled designs is clinical research. In: Medical uses of statistics. ed. by Bailar JC, Mosteller F, NEJM Books, Waltham, Ma, 1986, pp 67-90.

24. Packer M, Mellar J, Medina N, Gorlin R, Hermann RV. Rebound hemodynamic events after abrupt withdrawal of nitroprusside in patients with severe chronic heart failure. N Engl J Med 1979; 301: 1193-7.

25. Graham WG, Bradley DA. Efficacy of chest physiotherapy and intermittent positive- pressure breathing in the resolution of pneumonia. N Engl J Med 1978; 299,: 624-7.

26. Cleophas TJ. Adrenergic receptor agonist and antagonists in Raynaud's syndrome. Thesis, Nijmegen, Neth.,1983.

27. Cleophas TJ. Carryover effects in cardiovascular crossover studies: the standard and the clinical analysis. Angiology 1993; 44: 271-7.

CHAPTER 5

CLINICAL TRIALS: RELEVANCE OF CORRELATION BETWEEN TREATMENT RESPONSES

Background. Trials that do not allow to reject the null hypothesis of no treatment effect may have had an inappropriate design. Trials are virtually never assessed for correlation between responses to different treatment modalities.

Methods. Using a hypothetical example and several published studies we study the influence of correlation levels between treatment modalities on the sensitivity of testing.

Results. The level of correlation between responses to different treatment modalities is a major determinant of the sensitivity of both crossover and parallel group clinical trials.

Conclusions. It is extremely relevant to assess correlation levels between responses to the different treatment modalities of a trial a priori. If a negative correlation is anticipated a crossover design is likely to lack sensitivity. If a positive correlation is anticipated a parallel-group design would seem less appropriate because it would lack the extra sensitivity of accounting for the positive correlation. Both designs would seem suitable for approximately zero correlations (*e.g.* comparison vs baseline or vs placebo under the assumption that the number of placebo responders is negligible).

5.1   Introduction

In controlled clinical trials the new treatment may be a slight modification of the standard or be equivalent to it with the addition of a new component. In this situation there is a positive correlation between the new and the standard treatment: treatment 1 performs highly when treatment 2 does so. On the other hand, in trials with completely different treatments patients tend to fall apart into different populations: those who respond to treatment 1 and those who do to treatment 2. Patients with angina pectoris irresponsive to beta-blockers generally do respond either to calcium-antagonists or to nitroglycerines. Also hypertension, Raynaud's phenomenon, different types of cardiac arrhythmias, chronic obstructive pulmonary disease are known to be conditions where a non-response to a particular compound is frequently associated with an excellent response to a completely different compound. These are examples of situations in which a strong negative correlation may exist. This may even be so in crossover studies that otherwise are more likely to have a somewhat positive correlation because one subject is used for the comparison of two treatments. According to statisticians the issue of correlation is clinically relevant. For example, in a recent review of a Bayesian approach to crossover trials Grieve states that one should not comtemplate a crossover design at all, if there is any likelihood of correlation not being positive [1]. Clinicians and clinical pharmacologists, however, are generally unfamiliar with this issue and virtually never take it into account. The present paper tries to test two hypotheses. First, I hypothesized that the level of correlation between the responses to different treatment modalities is an important determinant of the sensitivity of crossover studies. Secondly, I hypothesized that this very mechanism may be responsible for several negative trials published so far. The first objective of this paper was to demonstrate to what extent the level of correlation influences the sensitivity of testing. The second was to develop a simple method that would enable to test a posteriori whether the cause of a negative result of a study is its particular level of correlation.

5.2   Levels of correlation and sensitivity of testing

In order to test the sensitivity of the differences in a paired group of data we use T-statistic under the assumption that our samples have a T-distribution. The larger the extent to which the T of the distribution to be tested differs from zero, the more sensitivity and power the statistical approach does provide. T is calculated according to

$$T = \frac{\text{mean}_{\text{test treatment}} - \text{mean}_{\text{reference treatment}}}{\text{se}_{\text{paired differences}}}$$

Obviously, the size of T is dependent not only on the treatment differences (differences between means) but also on their se (standard error). The larger se, the smaller the sensitivity and power of testing.

$$\text{se}_{\text{paired differences}} = \sqrt{[\sigma^2_{\text{test}} + \sigma^2_{\text{ref}} - 2\rho\sigma_{\text{test}}\,\sigma_{\text{ref}}]\,/\,n}$$

where σ_{test} and σ_{ref} are the standard deviations for the test treatment and reference treatment, respectively, and ρ is the correlation between the treatments.

Since standard deviations are non-negative entities, it is obvious that a positive correlation would give a smaller variance and hence a greater power for the paired design. A negative correlation would give less power for the paired design compared to the unpaired design while a zero correlation would result in the same power.

Suppose, we have a crossover study where $\sigma_{\text{test}} = \sigma_{\text{ref}}$, then the formula for se $_{\text{paired differences}}$
becomes $\sqrt{2\,\sigma^2\,(1-\rho)\,/\,n}$
It can be easily derived that se $= \sqrt{2\sigma^2\,/\,n}$ when $\rho = 0$.
When $\rho > 0$ se $< \sqrt{2\,\sigma^2\,/\,n}$.
When $\rho < 0$ se $> \sqrt{2\,\sigma^2\,/\,n}$.

Hypothetical example: in a trial of vasodilators for the treatment of Raynaud's phenomenon, 10 patients are treated with vasodilator one for 1 week and for a separate period of 1 week with vasodilator two. The data below show the numbers of Raynaud attacks/week. Although samples have identical means and σ's (25 ± 10 x-axis, 35 ± 10 y-axis), their correlation levels vary from -1 to +1. The major effect of correlation

levels on the statistical assessment can be readily understood when we look at the variances
of the paired differences.

CORRELATION:

$\rho = -1$	$\rho = 0$	$\rho = +1$
vasodilator	vasodilator	vasodilator
one two **paired differences**	one two **paired differences**	one two **paired differences**
50 10 40	50 40 10	15 10 5
45 15 30	45 35 10	25 15 10
45 15 30	45 35 10	30 15 15
40 20 20	40 30 10	30 20 10
35 25 10	35 25 10	35 25 10
35 25 10	35 10 25	35 25 10
30 30 0	30 15 15	40 30 10
30 35 -5	30 15 15	45 35 10
25 35 -10	25 20 5	45 35 10
15 40 -25	15 25 -10	50 40 10

mean

35 25 10	35 25 10	35 25 10
σ		
10 10 **20.4**	10 10 **8.8**	10 10 **2.4**

With a negative correlation, between-subject variation as estimated by σ is more than dou-
bled when we take the paired differences. With a positive correlation between-subject variability is largely removed when we do so. With a zero correlation the σ is in-between.
Although mean value of the paired differences is 10 in each of the three examples, their σ's
are largely different, 20.4, 8.8, and 2.4. The inversely proportional relationship between σ
and T's explains why the correlation level is a major determinant in the statistical analysis.

5.3   A simple test to check a posteriori whether the cause of a negative result is its level of correlation

The best method to check the level of correlation is to simply calculate the correlation-
coefficient. If, however, not all of the data are available, we have to look for an alternative.
Suppose, the result of a crossover study is negative. This may be due not only to (1)
small differences between treatments, (2) small sample size, and (3) large variances in
the trial, but also to (4) a negative correlation between treatments. We can account for
the size of (1), (2), and (3) by taking the division sum of difference of the means divided
by the se of the difference between the means. This value can be used as estimate of (1),

(2), and (3) and is actually identical to the T of an unpaired analysis of the data. Usually, it is smaller than the T of a paired analysis of the same data. It is not so, however, in the case of (4) a strong negative correlation.

$se_{\text{paired differences}} = \sqrt{[\sigma^2_{\text{test}} + \sigma^2_{\text{ref}} - 2\,\rho\sigma_{\text{test}}\,\sigma_{\text{ref}}]\,/\,n}$

$se_{\text{unpaired differences}} = \sqrt{[\sigma^2_{\text{test}} + \sigma^2_{\text{ref}}]\,/\,n}$

If we assume again that $\sigma_{\text{test}} = \sigma_{\text{ref}}$, then

$se_{\text{paired differences}} = \sqrt{2\,\sigma^2(1 - \rho)\,/\,n}$

$se_{\text{unpaired differences}} = \sqrt{2\,\sigma^2\,/\,n}$

This means that

$se_{\text{unpaired}} > se_{\text{paired}}$ when $\rho < 0$

$se_{\text{unpaired}} < se_{\text{paired}}$ when $\rho > 0$

This would mean that with a negative correlation the unpaired analysis of paired samples provides more sensitivity whereas the paired analysis does so with a positive correlation. With $\rho = 0$ both approaches offer similar sensitivity. Thus, we can make use of the unpaired approach assessment as a simple test for identifying negative correlations in paired comparisons a posteriori.

5.4   Review of published crossover studies with a presumably negative correlation

Figure 1 is an example of a published study with a strong negative correlation. The data are from the famous study of James Grizzle [2], one of the pioneers of crossover clinical trials. Two completely different compounds are tested for their abilities to increase hemoglobin. Treatment A is beneficial when treatment B is not so. On the other hand when treatment A fails,treatment B is to some degree successful. In this example, the paired approach offers little sensitivity (Figure 2). The unpaired approach (Figure 2: unpaired), however, did provide a significant result at p = 0.05. Obviously, this self-controlled study lacks power due to the negative correlation. Given that the existence of this potential problem has been recognized by statisticians [1], the issue raised by the current paper must be whether the problem is prevalent. In order to address this issue we analyzed 41 crossover studies published in the 1986 and 1987 volumes of The Lancet and The New England of Medicine. These studies have been reviewed by us for presence of carryover effects [3]. We took these studies because at that time the validity of crossover studies had been evaluated by the American Food and Drug Administration [4] and a number of statisticians [5-11]. In 6 of them (15%, Table I) either largely different compounds were compared, e.g., a ß-adrenergic agonist vs anticholinergic agent, an oral antidiabetic compound vs insulin, or otherwise completely different treatments such as different diets. The correlation between response to such different treatments is likely to be negative. The unpaired approach (Table I) confirms that this is so. It is consistently more sensitive than the paired approach. These studies are flawed and should have rather been performed as parallel group studies.

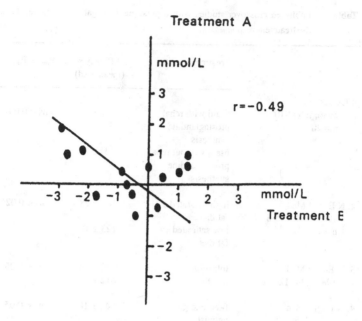

Figure 1. Graph of data from a published self-controlled study with
negative correlation [2].

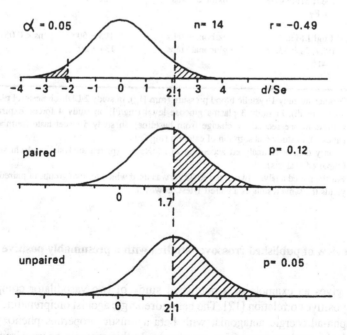

Figure 2. Statistical analysis of study from Figure 1 (T-statistic).

Table I. Published crossover studies with a presumably negative correlation between the treatment responses

	Treatment	Efficacy [0] (mean ± sd)	P_{paired} $P_{unpaired}$
1. Lancet 1986; i: 997-1001 n = 20	nsaid with renal prostaglandine synthesis	127 ± 3	ns < 0.001
	nsaid without renal prostaglandine synthesis	131 ± 3	
2. N Engl J Med 1986; 314: 745-8 n = 8	high saturated fat diet	163 ± 28	ns < 0.02
	low saturated fat diet	123 ± 18	
3. N Engl J Med 1986; 314: 1280-6	tolazolin	140 ± 34	ns < 0.05
	insulin	112 ± 15	
4. N Engl J Med 1986; 315: 735-9 N = 11	ß-adrenergic agonist	42 ± 18	ns < 0.05
	anticholinergic agent	25 ± 14	
5. N Engl J Med 1987; 316: 947-8 n = 89	new tabs	9/89 [*]	< 0.05 < 0.01
	oxidated tabs	22/89	
6. N Engl J Med 1987; 317: 532-6 n =16	carbonate tabs	195 ± 50 [#]	ns < 0.05
	gluconate tabs	134 ± 50	

[0] Denotes in study 1 systolic blood pressure (mm Hg), in study 2 LDL-cholesterol plasma level (mg/dl), in study 3 plasma glucose level (mg/dl), in study 4 forced expiratory volume in one second (% change from baseline), in study 5 sweet taste (number of patients), in study 6 absorption of calcium (mg %).

[*] Binary data were analyzed according to McNemar (paired analysis), and chi-square (unpaired analysis).

[#] For the paired analysis two-sided ANOVA was used which for two groups of paired data yields the same results as a paired T-test, however.

5.5   Review of published crossover studies with a presumably positive correlation

Figure 3 gives an example of a published study of two vasodilator compounds with a clearly positive correlation [12]. The beta-adrenergic agonist orciprenaline is compared to the alpha-adrenergic antagonist with beta-agonistic properties phenoxybenzamine. The graph shows a strong positive correlation. In this example an unpaired approach is likely to be weaker than a paired. Indeed, the analysis shows that the paired comparison provides sufficient sensitivity (Figure 4), whereas the unpaired did not. Table II shows the data of five self-controlled studies published in the 1986 and 1987 volumes of the New England Journal of Medicine and the Lancet. These studies compared equivalent compounds, e.g., two ß-adrenergic blockers, two cholesterol lowering compounds, etc. A positive correlation is anticipated. The unpaired approach (Table II) confirms that this is so. The paired approach is consistently more powerful than the unpaired. The studies are appropriately performed in the form of a self-controlled study. A parallel-group study would have lacked the extra sensitivity of accounting for the positive correlation.

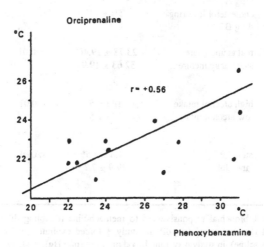

Figure 3. Graph of data from a published self-controlled study with positive correlation [12].

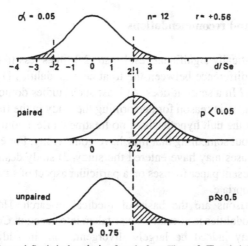

Figure 4. Statistical analysis of study from Figure 3 (T-statistic).

Table II. Published crossover studies with a presumably positive correlation between the treatment responses

	Treatment	Efficacy [0] (mean ± sd)	P_{paired}	$P_{unpaired}$
1. Lancet 1986; ii: 189-92 n = 6	Platelet activating factor its precursor	- 1.5 ± 1.0 + 0.2 ± 1.0	< 0.001	ns
2. Lancet 1986; ii: 740-1 n = 7	cholesterol lowering drug A cholesterol lowering drug B	42 ± 12 50 ± 12	< 0.05	ns
3. Lancet 1986; ii: 1419-21 n = 19	real acupuncture sham acupuncture	23.78 ± 19.46* 32.63 ± 19.99	< 0.01	ns
4. Lancet 1987; i: 647-52 n = 40	high alcohol intake low alcohol intake	143 ± 5 137 ± 5	< 0.01	ns
5. Lancet 1987; ii: 650-3 n = 20	atenolol labetalol	74.3 ± 4.5* 79.9 ± 7.2	< 0.01	ns

[0] Denotes in study 1 bronchial responsiveness to methacholine (doubling dilutions), in study 2 plasma level of HDL-cholesterol (mg/dl), in study 3 forced expiratory volume in one second (% change from baseline), in study 4 systolic blood pressure (mm Hg), in study 5 heart rate (bpm).
* For the paired analysis two-sided ANOVA was used which for two groups of paired data yields the same results as a paired T-test, however.

5.6   Conclusions and recommendations

Studies without statistically significant results are 2.3 times less likely to be published than those finding a difference between the treatment modalities [13]. Does this mean that they are a failure? In a sense it does. At least such studies do not confirm our prior beliefs, which was the main reason for performing the study in the first place. If the data do not allow to reject the null hypothesis of no treatment effect compared to control we have to think hard about something that may have gone wrong. For example, 1) samples were too small, 2) biases may have entered the study, 3) study designs may have been inappropriate. The present paper focuses on a particular aspect of study designs that may be sometimes inappropriate.

Treatment comparisons are the basis of medical research. However, correlation between treatment modalities is virtually never taken into account. Correlation in a treatment comparison may indeed be largely divergent, and, in addition, clinicians do frequently have arguments to estimate correlation levels a priori. To do so is extremely relevant because sensitivity and power of the statistical analysis will be largely determined by the very level of correlation. With a strong negative correlation a crossover design is likely to lack power. With a strong positive correlation a parallel study is less appropriate because it lacks the extra sensitivity of accounting for the positive correlation. Both designs should be suitable for approximately zero correlations. A comparison vs baseline or vs placebo may approximate a zero correlation, although not necessarily. The very existence of a consistent within patient placebo response is often the very factor which generates a somewhat positive correlation, making a self-controlled design ideal. All that it requires for this to work is that some patients should be placebo responders and that some should not. Study 5 from Table I suggests that the above mentioned overall conclusions can be drawn likewise when studies involve binary instead of continuous variables.

For the purpose of this paper T-statistic was used mainly. Other statistical methods for example analysis of variance or non-parametric statistic would probably yield similar results, however. Suppose analysis of variance would be performed of three paired samples. Sensitivity of testing is proportional to the size of

$$F = \frac{\text{Mean Square}_{\text{effect}}}{\text{Mean Square}_{\text{interaction}}}$$

If we take the positively correlated comparison from our hypothetical example twice and the negatively correlated comparison once, then

$$\text{Mean Square}_{\text{interaction}} = 2.4^2 + 2.4^2 + 20.4^2$$

If, however, we take the negatively twice and the positively correlated comparison once, then

$$\text{Mean Square}_{\text{interaction}} = 20.4^2 + 20.4^2 + 2.4^2$$

Obviously the denominator of the above division sum is largely determined by the correlation level while the numerator is not. The power of repeated measurement analysis of variance is thus largely influenced by level of correlation between treatment modalities similarly to paired T-statistic. A non-parametric analysis of the negatively correlated comparison of the hypothetical example using Mann-Whitney Rank-sum test yields a $p = 0.4$ (n.s.), while the positively correlated comparison yields a p of < 0.05. This is not too much of a surprise because this approach is strongly related to T-statistic in that the distribution of the sum of ranks looks a little bit like a T-distribution. It should be noticed that in the paired case you measure n patients twice and in the unpaired case you measure 2n patients once. Thus, if the cost per patients to a certain extent exceeds the cost per measurement, the paired design might be preferred if the correlation is zero or even modestly negative. It would, of course, be an overstatement to imply that the existence of a positive correlation is all that is required for crossover studies to be preferable to parallel group designs. There are many more potential drawbacks, e.g., carryover effects from one treatment period into the other, time effects due to spontaneously evolving symptoms, seasonal effects, given the longitude of such studies [3,14].

5.7   Conclusions

1. Correlation between treatment modalities in a controlled clinical trial is virtually never taken into account.
2. Clinicians do frequently have arguments to estimate correlation levels a priori.
3. To do so is extremely relevant because sensitivity and power of the statistical analysis will be largely determined by the correlation level. If a strong negative correlation is anticipated, a crossover design is likely to lack sensitivity and power, unless sample size compensates for this lack of power. If a positive correlation is anticipated, a parallel-group design would seem less appropriate because it would lack the extra sensitivity of accounting for the positive correlation. Both designs are suitable for a zero correlation (comparison versus placebo).
4. For those taking notice of a crossover study with a negative result, a simple test is presented that enables to detect negative correlations and can be used even when individual data of the samples are not available. For that purpose paired means are analyzed as though they are unpaired. When the unpaired assessment provides more sensitivity than the paired, correlation must be strong negative. The crossover design has then been inappropriately used and is responsible for the negative result of the study. When the unpaired assessment provides equal or less power, the correlation must be approximately zero or positive. The crossover design has been appropriately used.

Acknowledgment

The author is indebted to the editor and publisher of the European Journal of Clinical Pharmacology for granting permission to use parts of a paper previously published in the journal (1996; 50: 1-6).

References

1. Grieve AP. Bayesian analyses of two-treatment crossover studies. Stat Meth Med Res 1994; 3: 407-29.
2. Grizzle JE. The two-period change-over design and its use in clinical trials. Biometrics 2965; 22: 467-80.
3. Cleophas TJ. Testing crossover studies for carryover effects. Angiology 1989; 40: 287- 95.
4. Cornfield J, O'neill RT. Minutes of the Food and Drug Administration Advisory Committee Meeting, June, 23, 1976.
5. Wallenstein S, Fisher AC. The analysis of the two-period repeated measurements crossover design with application to clinical trials. Biometrics 1977; 33: 261-9.
6. Zimmermann H, Rahlfs V. Testing hypotheses in the two-period change-over with binary data. Biom J 1978; 20: 133-41.
7. Hills M, Armitage P. The two-period crossover clinical trial. Br J Clin Pharmacol 1979; 8: 7-20.
8. Brown BW. The crossover experiment for clinical trials. Biometrics 1980; 36: 69-79.
9. Presscott RJ. The comparison of success rates in crossover trials in the presence of an order effect. Appl Stat 1981; 30: 9-15.
10. Barker M, Hew RJ, Huitson A, Poloniecki J. The two-period crossover trial. Bull Appl Stat 1982; 9: 67-112.

11.Louis TA, Lavori PW, Bailar JC, Polansky M. Crossover and self-controlled designs in clinical research. N Engl J Med 1984; 310: 24-31.

12.Cleophas TJ, Fennis JFM, van 't Laar A. Alpha- and beta-blockade and beta-stimulation in Raynaud's syndrome. Angiology 1985; 36: 219-26.

13.Easterbrook PJ, Berlin JA, Gopalan R, Matthews Dr Publication bias in clinical research. Lancet 1991; 337: 867-72.

14.Cleophas TJ, Tavenier P. Fundamental issues of choosing the right type of trial. Am J Ther 1994; 1: 327-32.

CHAPTER 6

BETWEEN-GROUP DISPARITIES
IN DRUG RESPONSE

Background. In crossover clinical trials comparing completely different treatments patients tend to fall apart into different populations: those who respond better to treatment 1 and those who do so to treatment 2. The correlation between treatment response in such trials is negative. The current ANCOVA analysis for crossover studies does not allow for correlations being negative, and is, therefore, not adequate to test this kind of trials.
Objective of study. To study whether matrix algebra provides a more appropriate approach for this purpose.
Results and conclusions. Using a mathematical model as well as hypothesized examples I demonstrate that matrix algebra of 2 pairs of cells of the same order not only allows for negative correlations in a crossover design but also provides enough power to test both treatment and carryover effect.

6.1 Introduction

Following Grizzle and Brown [1,2], many workers [3-6] currently assume for the analysis of crossover studies the following statistical model based on analysis of covariance (ANCOVA):

$$y_{ijk} = \mu + \xi_{ij} + \pi_k + \Phi_l + \lambda_l + \in_{ijk}$$

where: y_{ijk} is the response for the jth subject in the ith sequence during the kth period
μ is the mean response
ξ_{ij} is the effect of the jth subject in the ith sequence
π_k is the effect of the kth period
Φ_l is the direct effect of the lth treatment
λ_l is the carryover effect of the lth treatment
$\in_{ijk}$ is the independent error term

$$\text{cov}(y_{ijk}, y_{ijk'}) = \quad \sigma^2_{\xi} + \sigma^2_{\epsilon} \qquad \text{if } k = k'$$
$$\sigma^2_{\xi} \qquad \text{if } k \text{ is not } k'$$

and

$$\text{corr}(y_{ij1}, y_{ij2}) = \sigma^2_{\xi} / (\sigma^2_{\xi} + \sigma^2_{\epsilon}) = \rho$$

The merit of this ANCOVA approach is that it enables in a fairly straightforward way to carry out an after-the-fact statistical adjustment on the data to equate on concomitant variables or covariates. However, the problems of this ANCOVA approach are:

1. that it does not allow for correlations being negative, because $\sigma^2_\xi / (\sigma^2_\xi + \sigma^2_\epsilon)$ simply cannot be negative,

2. that it fails to include a covariate related to differences in the populations under study.

On the one hand, in a treatment comparison the new treatment may be a slight modification of the standard or be equivalent to it with the addition of a new component. In this situation there is a positive correlation between the new and the standard treatment, i.e., treatment 1 will perform well when treatment 2 does so too. On the other hand, in trials with completely different treatments patients tend to fall apart into different populations : those who respond to treatment 1 and those who do so to treatment 2. Patients with angina pectoris unresponsive to beta-blockers generally do respond either to calcium channel blockers or to nitroglycerines. Also hypertension, Raynaud's phenomenon, different types of cardiac arrhythmias and chronic obstructive pulmonary disease are known to be conditions where a non-response to a particular conpound is frequently associated with an excellent response to a completely different compound. These are examples of situations in which a crossover study is likely to give rise to a strong negative correlation. This may even be so in spite of the likelihood in crossovers in general of a somewhat positive correlation because one subject is used for comparison of two treatments. The mechanism of between-group disparities has been well-recognized in clinical pharmacology, and is, in fact, the main reason that in treatment protocols the principle of stepped care is currently being replaced by individualized care [7]. The recognition of between-group disparities in drug response also implies that any mathematical approach for crossover studies should allow for correlations being negative, and that the above ANCOVA approach is not appropriate for that purpose. A more appropriate approach would be the application of basic matrix algebra in which 2x2 cells of the same order can be added or subtracted in a cell by cell manner. In the current paper it is studied whether this approach that unlike the ANCOVA allows for correlations being negative, provides adequate power to test both treatment and carryover effect.

6.2 Statistical model

According to Scheffé [8] the notation for a simple crossover study is:

	Period 1			Period 2	
	Treatment	Mean Efficacy		Treatment	Mean Efficacy
Group 1 n_1	1	$y_{1.1}$		2	$y_{1.2}$
Group 2 n_2	2	$y_{2.1}$		1	$y_{2.2}$

y_{ijk} = the response of the jth patient in the ith group in the kth period. We assume that $n_1 = n_2 = n$.

$Y_{i.k} = \Sigma y_{ijk}/n$

Also we assume :

1. that the samples have a normal distribution or a t-distribution,
2. that in a crossover without carryover effect the data of the second period are a true reflection of the first period because the two treatment groups are symmetric.

To test treatment effect(Φ)the sum of the results of treatment 1 is compared with the treatment 2 results($y_{1.1} + y_{2.2}$ vs $y_{1.2} + y_{2.1}$). To trace carryover effect (λ) the sum of the results in group 1 is compared with the group 2 results ($y_{1.1} + y_{1.2}$ vs $y_{2.1} + y_{2.2}$). To trace time effect (λ) the sum of the results in period 1 is compared with the period 2 results($y_{1.1} + y_{2.1}$ vs $y_{1.2} + y_{2.2}$).

The null-hypotheses that Φ, λ, and π are zero

$$\Phi \qquad [(y_{1.1} + y_{2.2})-(y_{1.2} + y_{2.1})] = 0$$
$$\lambda \qquad [(y_{2.1} + y_{2.2})-(y_{1.1} + y_{1.2})] = 0$$
$$\pi \qquad [(y_{1.1} + y_{2.1})-(y_{1.2} + y_{2.2})] = 0$$

should be slightly remodeled into

$$\Phi \qquad [(y_{1.1} - y_{1.2})-(y_{2.1} - y_{2.2})] = 0$$
$$\lambda \qquad [(y_{2.1} + y_{2.2})-(y_{1.1} + y_{1.2})] = 0$$
$$\pi \qquad [(y_{1.1} - y_{1.2})+(y_{2.1} - y_{2.2})] = 0$$

In this way 2x2 paired cells can be adequately added or subtracted in a cell by cell manner.

These null hypotheses can be tested,for example,by t-statistic or one-way analysis of variance(ANOVA). The larger the extent to which the t or F value of our distribution differs from zero, the more sensitivity and power the statistical approach does provide.

$$t = \frac{d}{SE} \text{ (or one-way ANOVA, F value)}$$

where d is Φ, λ, or π, and SE is their standard error.

SE is calculated by use of the standard formulas for the variance (σ^2) of paired and unpaired sums and differences.

$\sigma^2_{paired\ sums} = \sigma_1^2 + \sigma_2^2 + 2\rho\sigma_1\sigma_2$
$\sigma^2_{paired\ differences} = \sigma_1^2 + \sigma_2^2 - 2\rho\sigma_1\sigma_2$
$\sigma^2_{unpaired\ sums} = \sigma_1^2 + \sigma_2^2$
$\sigma^2_{unpaired\ differences} = \sigma_1^2 + \sigma_2^2$

We assume that $\sigma = \sigma_{Y1.1} = \sigma_{Y1.2} = \sigma_{Y2.1} = \sigma_{Y2.2}$ = standard deviation of the samples in each of the cells, and that $\rho = \rho_{Y1.1\ vs\ Y1.2} = \rho_{Y2.1\ vs\ Y2.2}$ = correlation coefficient between the samples of each of the two paired cells.

Then

$$\sigma^2_{\Phi} = 2\,(2\sigma^2)\,(1 - \rho)$$
$$\sigma^2_{\lambda} = 2\,(2\sigma^2)\,(1 + \rho)$$
$$\sigma^2_{\pi} = 2\,(2\sigma^2)\,(1 - \rho)$$

Because $n_1 = n_2 = n$ we now can calculate the SE's as follows:

$SE_{\Phi} \quad = \sqrt{4\sigma^2\,(1 - \rho)\,(1/2n + 1/2n)}$
$\qquad\quad = \sqrt{4\sigma^2\,(1 - \rho)\,/\,n}$

and accordingly

$SE_{\lambda} \quad = \sqrt{4\sigma^2(1 + \rho)\,/\,n}$
$SE_{\pi} = \sqrt{4\sigma^2(1-\rho)\,/\,n}$

Suppose $\lambda = \Phi$ and $\rho = 0$, then $t_\lambda = t_\Phi$. In this situation the powers to test carryover and treatment effect are equal.

If $\lambda = \Phi$ and $\rho > 0$ then $t_\lambda < t_\Phi$

If $\lambda = \Phi$ and $\rho < 0$ then $t_\lambda > t_\Phi$

So, the powers of testing are largely dependent on the correlation between treatment modalities ρ. Whenever $\rho > 0$ we soon will have much more power to test treatment effect than carryover effect of similar size. We should add that in practice $\sigma_{Y1.2}$ may be somewhat larger than $\sigma_{Y1.1}$, because the larger the data the larger the variances. If, $e.g.$, $\sigma_{Y1.2}$ is 10% larger than $\sigma_{Y1.1}$, ρ will change from > 0 to > 0.05. So, in this situation the level of positive correlation required tends to rise.

If the situation allows to assume that the reference treatment in the trial is inert, it will not usually cause carryover effect, and consequently we, thus, will be able to account for carryover effect only in the group that received the active treatment after the inert treatment. Assuming that treatment 1 is inert then we will have to account for carryover effect in group 2 only and the appropriate analysis for carryover effect in this situation thus becomes

λ $(y_{2.2}-y_{1.1}) = 0$

SE is calculated by use of the formula for unpaired differences

σ_λ^2 $= 2\sigma^2$

SE_λ $= \sqrt{2\sigma^2(1/n + 1/n)}$

SE_λ $= \sqrt{4\sigma^2/n}$

Again,   if $\lambda = \Phi$,   and $\rho = 0$ then $t_\lambda = t_\Phi$

       if $\lambda = \Phi$ and $\rho > 0$ then $t_\lambda < t_\Phi$

       if $\lambda = \Phi$ and $\rho < 0$ then $t_\lambda > t_\Phi$

Time effect (π) is considered to influence the data of the two treatments in a similar way, and its influence on treatment differences is, thus, negligible.

	Period 1		Period 2	
	Treatment	Mean response	Treatment	Mean response
Group 1	1	$y_{1.1}$	2	$y_{1.2} + \frac{1}{2}\pi$
Group 2	2	$y_{2.1}$	1	$y_{2.2} + \frac{1}{2}\pi$

Under the assumption $\lambda = 0$ we have Φ $= (y_{1.1}-y_{1.2}-\frac{1}{2}\pi)-(y_{2.1}-y_{2.2}-\frac{1}{2}\pi)$

                                                  $= y_{1.1}-y_{1.2}-y_{2.1} + y_{2.2}$

While the estimate of time or period effect may be relevant to clinicians its size apparently does not influence the analysis of the treatment data, and so it does not have to be taken into account.

6.3   Hypothetical examples, power analysis

The power of testing treatment effect is, thus, heavily dependent on the variances of
the paired differences. This can be illustrated by the example from Figure 1. It shows
how levels of correlation between two treatment modalities influence the variances of
paired differences opposedly. In the case of a negative correlation the SE of the paired
differences largely outnumbers the SE of the positive correlation situation, while
the zero-correlation-SE is in between. This is, of course, the main reason that finding
a significant difference between two samples with a positive correlation is a lot easier
than doing so with a negative. Suppose, we have 3 crossovers with the data of Figure 1
in Group 1 and with Group 2 a true reflection of Group 1.

	Period 1		Period 2	
	Treatment	Mean Response	Treatment	Mean Response
Group 1 n=10	1 Y1.1	35 ± 10	2 Y1.2	25 ± 10
Group 2 n=10	2 Y2.1	25 ± 10	1 Y2.2	35 ± 10

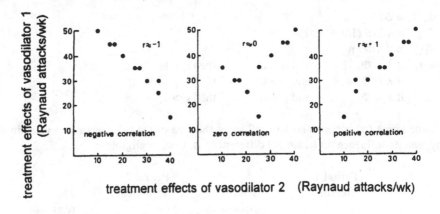

Figure 1. Individual values of paired observations with similar group means, n's and SD's
(vasodilator 1   35 ± 10,   vasodilator 2   25 ± 10).
negative correlation   ($\rho \cong -1$):   SE paired differences 6.8
zero correlation   ($\rho \cong 0$):   SE paired differences 2.9
positive correlation   ($\rho \cong +1$):   SE paired differences 0.8

In the given example improvement is measured by the number of Raynaud
attacks/wk. Vasodilator 2 is more efficient than vasodilator 1, because we have less
attacks. Suppose, this result causes a physical carryover effect in Group 2 from period 1

into period 2. Then, the mean value at $y_{2.2}$ changes from 35 into 35-λ, where λ = mean value of carryover effect in Group 2 of the trial. If for the purpose of this particular example we assume that the variance of λ is zero, it can be simply subtracted from the paired differences of the groups without influencing their SE's. It does not invalidate the overall conclusions of the procedure because any variance larger than zero has to be added to the variances already in the study, thus, further reducing the power of testing.

So, the assumption produces the largest powers for the given data. Calculations are carried out by paired and unpaired t-statistic and power is approximated from the equation POWER = 1 - ß = 1 - prob [Z ≤ (t¹ - t)] where Z represents the standardized value for the differences between two means and t¹ represents the upper critical value of t for the given degrees of freedom and α has been specified (treatment effect α = 0.05, carryover effect α = 0.10 according to Grizzle (1). In Figure 2 power graphs are drawn of tests for treatment and carryover effects of the three crossover situations from Figure 1 with the variable λ added. First, there are three power curves of treatment effect for the three correlation situations. As λ increases, all three gradually come down. The negative correlation curve is the first to do so. Consequently, this situation has generally little power of rightly coming to the right conclusion. At λ = 10, when treatment effect is equal to carryover effect, there is less than 30% power left. It means we have a more than 70% chance that treatment effect is erroneously unobserved in this study. Considering that a power of approximately 80% is required for reliable testing, we cannot test carryover here in a sensitive manner. The zero and positive correlation situations provide essentially more power.

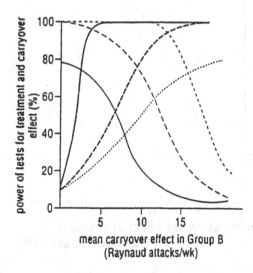

Figure 2. Power graphs of tests for treatment effect (slope downwards) and carryover effect(slope upwards) of the three crossover situations from Figure 1 with the variable λ (mean carryover effect in group 2) added.

———————————————— $\rho \cong -1$

— — — — — — — — $\rho \cong 0$

------------------------------ $\rho \cong +1$

There are also three power curves of carryover effect for the three correlation situations. The negative correlation curve provides essentially better power than the zero and positive correlation curves do. This example shows that strong positive correlations leave little power to test carryover effect. It also shows that strong negative correlations produce excessive power to test carryover effect.

Figure 3 gives the alternative approach where carryover effect is tested according to the one-group carryover principle. In this approach the three different correlation situations have one and the same carryover curve because the unpaired comparison for carryover has identical means, SD's, and n's, and is, thus, not influenced by different levels of correlation. It is actually the same curve as the λ=0 curve from Figure 2. Its power increases with increase of λ. At λ = 10 when treatment effect is equal to carryover effect, it is about 80%.

The latter approach should be performed instead of the former whenever modalities of treatment allow to do so. This is because it both offers less power with negative correlations and more power with positive correlations. In so doing it one time prevents the detection of small and clinically irrelevant carryover effects, and one time the detection of small and clinically unimportant treatment effects.

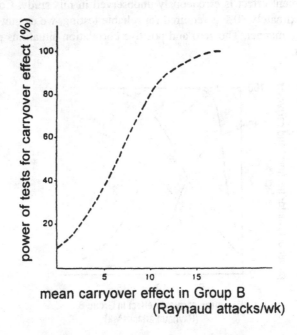

mean carryover effect in Group B
(Raynaud attacks/wk)

Figure 3. Power graph of tests for carryover effect of the three crossover situations from Figure 1 with the variable λ (mean carryover effect in group 2) added.
The graph displays carryover effect irrespective of size of ρ (one-group carryover effect analysis).

6.4 Discussion

Crossover studies are routinely used in clinical research. For example not less than 22% of the double-blind placebo-controlled hypertension trials published in 1993 were crossover [9,10]. A major advantage of the crossover design is that it eliminates between-subject variability of symptoms.

However, problems include the occurrence of carryover and time effects, and the fact that the design itself offers little power to test such effects. Power of testing such effects is enhanced by use of ANCOVA which is able to test treatment, carryover and time effects simultaneously [3-6]. ANCOVA in its current form does not allow, however, for correlations being negative which is an important possibility in studies comparing completely different treatments. Adding another covariate to adjust this flaw weakens the ANCOVA, and makes it hardly testable. An alternative approach is the classic two-stage analysis in which carryover and time effects are tested first and treatment effect second. Power of this approach is enhanced when data are analyzed by use of matrix algebra. Data are analyzed in the form of 2x2 cells of the same order, that are added or subtracted in a cell by cell manner.

The alternative analysis for crossover studies as presented in this paper includes the following steps:
1. Carryover and treatment effects in a crossover study are tested by use of matrix algebra according to which 2 pairs of cells of the same order are added or subtracted.
2. A one-group analysis for carryover effect is performed whenever the clinical situation allows to do so. It generally offers a more adequate power to test the data.
3. Thile the estimate of time effects may be relevant to clinicians its size does not influence the estimate of the treatment effects, and, therefore, does not have to be taken into account in the analysis of the treatment data.
4. In crossover trials with a zero or positive correlation small carryover effects hardly reduce the power of demonstrating a treatment effect. It does make sense, nonetheless, to test for carryover effect the group that received the effective compound first. If such testing is positive, a parallel-group analysis of period 1 of the trial can effectively be used for demonstrating a treatment effect. In case of a significant carryover effect in group 2 a parallel-group analysis of period 1 will provide a significant test as well, and it will do so at the same or even at a higher level of significance than the test for carryover effect. This is because when carryover effect is maximal, the mean response in period 2 group 2 being $y_{2.2}$ equals $y_{2.1}$. The between-group difference between $y_{2.1}$ and $y_{1.1}$ in period 1 will, therefore, be at least as large as the difference between $y_{2.2}$ and $y_{1.1}$ but probably larger. Therefore, no further test for treatment effect seems to be required in this situation and the data of period 2 could be disregarded. If we wish to enhance the power of testing this situation even so, we could perfectly well make use of the unbiased period-2-data of group 1 using a weighting procedure [11].

Acknowledgement

The author is indebted to the editor and publisher of the European Journal of Clinical Chemistry/Clinical Biochemistry for granting permission to use parts of a paper previously published in the journal (1997; 35: 775-9).

References

1. Grizzle JE. The two-period change-over design and its use in clinical trials. Biometrics 1965; 22: 469-80.
2. Brown BW. The crossover experiment for clinical trials. Biometrics 1980; 36: 69-79.
3. Grieve A. A bayesian analysis of the two- period crossover design for clinical trials. Biometrics 1985; 41: 979-90.
4. Willan AR,Pater JL. Carryover and the two- period crossover clinical trial. Biometrics 1986; 42: 593-9.
5. Freeman PR. The performance of the two- stage analysis of two-treatment, two-period crossover trials. Stat Med 1989; 8: 1421- 32.
6. Fleiss JA. A critique of recent research on the two-treatment crossover design. Control Clin Trials 1989; 10: 237-44.
7. Nies AS, Spielberg SP. Individualization of drug therapy. In: Hardman JL *et al.*, editors. Goodman and Gilman's Pharmacological Basis of Therapeutics. New York: McGraw- Hill, 1996, pp 43-63.
8. Scheffé H. Mixed models. In: Scheffé H, editor. The analysis of variance. New York, Wiley & Sons, 1959, pp 261-91.
9. Cleophas TJ. Clinical trials : relevance of correlation between treatment responses. Eur J Clin Pharmacol 1996; 50: 1-6.
10. Jackson PR,Yeo WW,Cleophas TJ. Crossover trials. Br J Clin Pharmacol 1996; 42: 399-404.
11. Cleophas TJ. Crossover studies :a modified analysis with more power. Clin Pharmacol Ther 1993; 53: 515-20.

CHAPTER 7
SPECIFIC PROBLEMS WITH TRIALS OF
CHRONIC DISEASES

In spite of rather negative publicity on the crossover/self-controlled design for clinical trials in the early 80's the Lancet and the New England Journal of Medicine published 41 such studies soon afterwards. Using these studies as examples I try to give an overview of major advantages and disadvantages of crossover and parallel group studies. Strengths of the crossover versus parallel design include: (1) elimination of between-subject variability of symptoms, (2) no need for large samples, (3) fewer ethical problems, (4) the test-persons are able to express their preference for one of the compounds being given. Weaknesses include: (1) carryover effect from one treatment period into the other, (2) time effect due to spontaneously evolving symptoms in a lengthy trial. The crossover/self-controlled design although routinely used for all types of therapies in phase I/II studies cannot be used in phase III/IV studies otherwise than for symptomatic treatments of stable disease. Treatments of chronic diseases are directed primarily to the relief of persistent symptoms rather than the cure of a rapidly evolving symptomatology. These very aspects make them particularly suitable for crossover/self-controlled studies. All of the advantages are involved while the disadvantages are not relevant. Recent statistical reports support these findings. Clinical practitioners will find it useful to consider the suitability of the trial design for the condition under study when assessing the practical importance of published reports of clinical trials.

7.1   Introduction

So many unpredictable variables may play a role in clinical trials of medical treatments, that, by now, a trial without controls has become almost inconceivable. The following methods [1] are routinely used:
1) A single patient receives both a new treatment and a standard treatment or placebo (crossover or self-controlled design).
2) For every patient given a new treatment, a control patient is given a placebo or standard treatment (parallel group design).

The advantage of a crossover/self-controlled design is that between-subject variability of symptoms in a disease is reduced, because every patient serves as his/her own control. The disadvantage is, however, the possibility of carryover effect: if the effect of the first treatment period carries on into the second, then it influences the response to the second treatment. This means that the design can hardly be used except for testing short-term effects of drugs or for symptomatic treatment of chronic stable disease. Even then, small curative or time effects may substantially bias the data, as in wound healing by vasodilators [2]. During the late 70's and early 80's, the American Food and Drug Administration [3] and many statisticians [4-10] discussed this point and discouraged use of crossover/self-controlled designs where an unbiased estimation of treatment effect is required. In spite of this rather negative publicity, the Lancet and the New England Journal of Medicine still published 41 crossover studies in 1986-7. Using these publications as examples, I summarize major advantages and disadvantages of crossover and parallel group investigations. Secondly, I assess the influence of the stage of the study and the type of disease on the choice of design. And thirdly, I evaluate recent statistical papers on the subject to determine the role of crossover/self-controlled designs in current medical research.

This review is not intended for those who perform clinical trials since for them, this material is well-known. Instead, we address those in clinical practice who depend on reports of clinical trials when making clinical decisions. Awareness of the weaknesses of clinical trials is especially important to them.

7.2   Published clinical trials

In 1986-7 The Lancet and The New England Journal of Medicine published 41 crossover studies (Table I) [11-50]. The number of parallel group studies in the same issues was 192. Not less than 18% of all clinical trials were crossover, indicating that the crossover design plays an important role in medical research. An advantage of a crossover design is that it provides an opportunity to compare different treatment periods with each other and to conclude from that whether a time effect (the disease spontaneously evolves by time) or a carryover effect is apparent [51]. Fifteen of the 41 published papers (36%) were studied for these effects. Accounting for such effects is impossible in parallel group designs [52]. All of the crossover studies were phase III/IV, involving therapies designed to treat chronic stable diseases or recurrent conditions.

Although 40% of the papers dealt with cardiovascular conditions, there were papers about a wide variety of other chronic conditions.

7.3   Strengths and weaknesses of the two designs

7.3.1   STRENGTHS OF CROSSOVER VERSUS PARALLEL-GROUP STUDIES

1. Between-subject variability of symptoms may be large in chronic debilitating conditions and pain syndromes (for example, neurologic conditions, rheumatoid arthritis, angina pectoris). A large between-subject variability reduces the statistical power of parallel-group studies and is eliminated by the use of a crossover design.
2. With a crossover design there is no need for large samples. Every patient serves as his/her own control. This is why only half of the numbers of patients are required compared to an equivalent parallel-group investigation. This aspect is particularly important to investigators of rare diseases, for example, paralysis due to cobra bite, spastic torticollis, hypogonadism. The numbers of patients studied in Table I were small indeed. They varied

from 6 to 32 (mean value 12). Even the studies that involved 10 patients or less could frequently reject the null hypothesis with a power of approximately 77% or more ($p < 0.01$), which is in general a good power to aim at.

3. With a crossover none of the patients has to use a placebo throughout the trial because treatments are crossed half-way.

This is the reason that ethicists frequently do have less concern with crossover than with parallel group designs, although for the study of chronic psychiatric conditions a crossover design may still be unethical [53]. This point is particularly relevant to potentially life-threatening conditions(for example, cardiac conditions, COPD, paralysis). An observational study (case-control, cohort) may raise even fewer ethical problems than a crossover (the treatment group is compared to an untreated control group or to the entire population instead of a placebo group). However, it frequently cannot give a definitive answer because the treatment group differs from its controls in many more ways than in clinical trials.

4. A crossover design enables the test-persons to express directly their preference for one of the compounds being given. This point is less relevant for the study of objective variables, for example, blood pressure, temperature, blood flow. However, for the study of pain syndromes (for example, dysmenorrhoea, heart burn, angina pectoris) it provides valuable extra information.

The above points are the main reasons that clinicians feel attracted to crossover studies. As for statisticians, an additional advantage is that the positive correlation between observations for one subject reduces variances of a comparative study.

7.3.2 WEAKNESSES OF CROSSOVER VERSUS PARALLEL-GROUP STUDIES

1. If a patient is cured by a treatment, he/she cannot be used again as a test-person in the next period of a trial. Even with non-curative treatments small curative effects may sometimes occur, for example, wound healing by vasodilators. This points directly to the weakest part of crossover studies. If such aN effect of an active treatment carries on in the next treatment period, then it will influence the response to the latter period. Interposing a wash-out period between the two treatment periods cannot entirely prevent this happening. What follows is that the difference between period 1 and 2 is minimized and that the risk of erroneously accepting the null hypothesis of no difference between active treatment and placebo (type II error) is enhanced. If it does not come to that, then there is an increased probability that the active treatment will be underestimated when compared to placebo [2].

2. For a crossover study a relatively stable chronic condition is required. For example, Raynaud's phenomenon is essentially more symptomatic in winter than in summer. A trial that tests vasodilators needs to be completed, therefore, in one winter, because in spring symptoms often improve spontaneously. This point is even more a problem as crossover studies generally take longer than equivalent parallel group studies due to their more than one treatment period principle. In order to reduce the risk of this so called time effect, some investigators favor the use of relatively short periods of treatment and subsequently apply surrogate endpoints to estimate the supposed long-term effects.

Doing so is, however, highly speculative. Short-term effects may not reveal adequately the more important long-term effects [54]. For example, many antihypertensive drugs do not reduce peripheral resistance until treatment has been in progress for several months. In such situations long-term studies are indispensable, using either crossover or parallel designs.

Table I. Crossover studies of therapies designed to treat chronic diseases published in the Lancet and the New England of Medicine in 1986-7 (41 papers)

Disease Type	Condition Studied	References
Gynaecology	dysmenorrhoea	11
Neurology	tardive dyskinesia	12
	spastic torticollis	13
	paralysis due to cobra bite	14
	Alzheimer	15
Cardiovascular	cardiac failure	16-19
Disease	angina pectoris	20,21
	Raynaud's phenomenon	22
	hypertension	23-33
Pulmonology	chronic obstructive pulmonary disease	34-36
Otorhinolaryngology	allergic rhinitis	37
	acute allergy (atopy)	38
Gastroenterology	malabsorption syndromes	39, 40
	hyperacidity syndromes	41, 42
Metabolic Diseases	hyperlipemia	43, 44
	pathologic obesity	45
	osteoporosis	46
Endocrinology	hypogonadism	47
	diabetes mellitus	48
Rheumatology	rheumatoid arthritis	49
Environmental Diseases	jet lag	50

How, in general, did the Lancet and the New England Journal of Medicine papers handle the problems of carryover and time effect? On the one hand 26/41 papers (63%) did not even mention whether they considered the possibility of such effects. Of the remaining 15 papers only 6 (15%) tested the data for such effects, and 3 of them, actually, found such an effect. The other 9 papers only mentioned that they considered the possibility without any further attempt to evaluate it. On the other hand, the indication for a crossover design seemed appropriate without exception. The design was used for chronic stable conditions and symptomatic treatments.

If a carryover or time effect is expected, a parallel group design is essential. This implies that for acute diseases and curative treatments the crossover design is largely unsuitable. Perhaps for the purpose of acute experiments, in very early stages of the development of new compounds this is not so. In this outline the n = 1 trial takes a separate place: a single patient is given in a double-blind fashion two or more therapies. As a matter of fact, we are not dealing with purely scientific research here, but with the determination of an optimal therapy for an individual patient [55].

7.4   Stage of study and the type of trial

In phase I/II trials small groups of volunteers or patients are tested for short-term effects of new drugs, for example, by means of dose response and dose titration studies. For this purpose, a crossover/self-controlled design is frequently used, which tests a group of subjects more than once. This is so regardless of whether a symptomatic or curative treatment is involved. In phase III/IV trials the situation is different. Such trials are generally of longer duration than phase I/II studies. It follows that for the study of acute diseases that must be cured, only parallel group studies can be applied. Some statisticians and the FDA have even pointed out that in all phase III/IV trials a parallel group design should be applied and there is basically no place for self-controlled/crossover designs here [3-10]. In spite of this, 41 crossovers were published in the Lancet and the New England Journal of Medicine afterwards that were phase III/IV and involved chronic conditions. The absence of phase I/II studies may be due to the publishing policy of the journals. It may be relevant at this point to make a distinction between two different types of phase IV studies, (1) investigations among large numbers of patients in parallel groups issued for the detection of rare side effects of a new treatment rather than its efficacy (we exclude the so called promotional phase IV studies) and (2) large-scale trials for the purpose of the determination of the ultimate place of a new treatment compared to standard or placebo. Because common symptomatology is involved in the latter instance and not so much rare side-effects, this type of phase IV study could gain in statistical power by a crossover design, because between-subject variability of symptoms is eliminated. In addition, the costs of such research may be easier to contain because fewer test-subjects are needed and ethical committees will approve such trials more readily because seriously ill patients need not be treated with a placebo or an in efficient compound throughout the trial. One might contend, therefore, that for studying chronic diseases, for which treatment is directed primarily to relief of persistent symptoms phase III/IV crossover studies do have a place. All of the advantages are involved, while the disadvantages are not relevant.

7.5   More recent statistical papers on the subject

In the late 80's and early 90's statisticians realized that no help regarding the problem of carryover effect was to be expected from the data. They considered the need for clinical arguments such as appropriate indications. Freeman [56] and Woods *et al.* [57] rejected the standard two-stage analysis of crossover studies where carryover is tested firstly and treatment effect secondly. They recommended the bayesian approach of an a priori knowledge of carryover, that was first described by Grieve [53]. Although Willan [58] assumed that appropriate indications would sufficiently curtail carryover and time effects, Fleiss [59] recommended testing this assumption by some kind of preliminary test. Apparently, modern statisticians no longer categorically reject the crossover design. They also have increasingly come to appreciate clinical arguments. In addition, Cleophas described some improvements of the standard mathematical approach which displayed both more sensitivity and power than the standard approach did thus far [60]. Most recently, the biostatistician Senn [61] wrote a substantial book on the subject concluding that there is definitely a place for the crossover/self-controlled design although both the design and the analysis should depend not only on the statistical principle but also on "what else we know".

7.6   Conclusions

Strengths of the crossover versus parallel design include: (1) elimination of between-subject variability of symptoms, (2) no need for large samples, (3) fewer ethical problems, (4) the test-persons are able to express their preference for one of the compounds being given. Weaknesses include: (1) carryover effect from one treatment period into the other, (2) time effect due to spontaneously evolving symptoms in a lengthy trial. The crossover/self-controlled design although routinely used for all types of studies in phase I/II research cannot be used in phase III/IV studies otherwise than for symptomatic treatments of stable disease. Treatments of chronic diseases are directed primarily to the relief of persistent symptoms rather than the cure of a rapidly evolving symptomatology. These very aspects make them particularly suitable for crossover/self-controlled studies. All of the advantages are involved while the disadvantages are not relevant. Recent statistical reports support these findings.

Acknowledgement

The author is indebted to the editor and publisher of the Journal of Clinical Pharmacology for granting permission to use parts of a paper previously published in the journal (1995; 35: 594-8).

References

1. Moses LE. Statistical concepts fundamental to investigations. N Engl J Med 1985; 312: 890-7.
2. Cleophas TJ. Underestimation of treatment effect in crossover trials. Angiology 1990; 41: 855-64.
3. Cornfield J, O'neill RT. Minutes of the Food and Drug Administration Advisory Committee Meeting, June, 23, 1976.
4. Wallenstein S, Fisher AC. The analysis of the two-period repeated measurements crossover design with application to clinical trials. Biometrics 1977; 33: 261-9.
5. Zimmermann H, Rahlfs V. Testing hypotheses in the two-period change-over with binary data. Biom J 1978; 20: 133-41.
6. Hills M, Armitage P. The two-period crossover clinical trial. Br J Clin Pharmacol 1979; 8: 7-20.
7. Brown BW. The crossover experiment for clinical trials. Biometrics 1980; 36: 69-79. 8. Presscott RJ. The comparison of success rates in crossover trials in the presence of an order effect. Appl Stat 1981; 30: 9-15.
9. Barker M, Hew RJ, Huitson A, Poloniecki J. The two-period crossover trial. Bull Appl Stat 1982; 9: 67-112.
10.Louis TA, Lavori PW, Bailar JC, Polansky M. Crossover and self-controlled designs in clinical research. N Engl J Med 1984; 310: 24-31.
11.Reginald PW, Beard RW, Kooner JS, Mathias CJ, Samarage SU. Intravenous dihydroergotamine to relieve pelvic congestion with pain in young women. Lancet 1987; 2: 351-3.
12.Lohr JB, Cadet JH, Lohr MA, Jeste DV, Wyatt RJ. Alpha-tocopherol in tardive dyskinesia. Lancet 1987; 1: 913-4.
13.Tsui JKC, Eisen A, Stoessl AJ, Calne S, Calne DB. Double-blind study of botulinum toxin in spasmodic torticollis. Lancet 1986; 2: 245-8.
14.Watt G, Theakston RDG, Hayes CG, Yambao ML, Sangalung R, Ranoa C, Alquizalus E, Warrell DA. Positive response to edrophonium in patients with neurotoxic envenoming by cobras (Naja Philippinensis). N Engl J Med 1986; 315: 1444-8.
15.Koopmans W, Majovski LV, Marsh GM, Tachiki K, Kling A. Oral tetrahydroaminoacridine in long-term treatment of senile dementia, Alzheimer type. N Engl J Med 1986; 315: 1241-5.
16.Cowley AJ, Stainer K, Wynne RD, Rowley JM, Hampton JR. Symptomatic assessment of patients with heart failure: double-blind comparisons of increasing doses of diuretics and captopril in moderate heart failure. Lancet 1986; 2: 770-2.
17.Crozier IG, Nichols MG, Ikran H, Epinder EA, Gomez HJ, Warner BJ. Haemodynamic effects of atrial peptide infusion in heart failure. Lancet 1986; 2: 1242-5.
18.Kirch W, Halabi H, Ohnhaus EE. Negative inotropic effects of famotidine. Lancet 1987; 2: 684-5.
19.Richardson A, Bayliss J, Scriben AJ, Parameschar J, Poole-Wilson PA, Sutton GE. Double-blind comparison of captopril alone against frusemide plus amiloride in mild heart failure. Lancet 1987; 2: 709-11.
20.Hasegawa GR, Gabin SS. Subjective indicators of nitroglycerin potency. N Engl J Med 1987; 316: 947-8.
21.Parker JO, Farrell B, Lahey KA, Moe G. Effects of intervals between doses on the development of tolerance to isosorbide dinitrate. N Engl J Med 1987; 316: 1440-4.
22.Ernst E, Matrai A, Kollar L. Placebo- controlled, double-blind study of haemodilution in peripheral arterial disease. Lancet 1987; 1: 1449-52.
23.Puddy IB. Pressor effect of alcohol. Lancet 1985; 2: 1119-21.
24.Dunn JM, Groth PE, de Simone A. Once-daily propranolol. Lancet 1985; 2: 1183-4.
25.Hauger JH. Comparison of sublingual captopril and nifedipine. Lancet 1986; 1: 219-20.
26.Bowler GMR, Galloway DW, Meiklejohn BH, Macintyre CCA. Sharp fall in blood pressure after injection of heparin containing chlorbutol. Lancet 1986; 1: 848-9.
27.Peltola H, Heinomen OP. Frequency of true adverse reactions to measles-mumps-rubella vaccine. Lancet 1986; 1: 939-42.
28.Wong DG, Spence JD, Lanki L, Freeman D, McDonald A. Effect of non-steroidal anti-inflammatory drugs on control of hypertension by beta-blockers and diuretics. Lancet 1986; 1: 997-1001.
29.Nelson L, Jennings GL, Esler MD, Korner PJ. Effect of changing levels of physical activity on blood pressure and haemodynamics in essential hypertension. Lancet 1986; 2: 473-9.
30.Woo J, Woo KS, Vallance Owen J. Captopril versus hydrochlorothiaizde/triamterene in mild to moderate hypertension in the elderly. Lancet 1986; 2: 924.

31. Wall-Manning HJ, Paulin JM. Sodium supplements, blood pressure, and calcium channel blocking drugs. Lancet 1987; 1: 1370.

32. Roberts DH, Tsao Y, McLoughlin GA, Breckenridge A. Placebo-controlled comparison of captopril, atenolol,labetalol, and pindolol in hypertension complicated by intermittent eladication. Lancet 1987; 2: 650-3.

33. Waeber B, Scherrer U, Petrillo A, Bidiville J, Nussberger J, Waeber G. Are some hypertensive patients overtreated. Lancet 1987; 2: 732-4.

34. Easton PA, Jadue C, Dingra S, Anthonisen NR. A comparison of the broncho dilating effects of a beta-2 adrenergic agent (albuterol) and an anticholinergic agent (ipratropium bromide), given by aerosol alone or in sequence. N Engl J Med 1986; 315: 735-9.

35. Cuss FM, Dixon CM, Barnes PJ. Effects of inhaled platelet activating factor on pulmonary function and bronchial responsiveness in man. Lancet 1986; 2: 189- 92.

36. Fung KP, Wun Chow OK, So SY. Attenuation of exercise-induced astma by acupuncture. Lancet 1986; 2: 1419-21.

37. Pipkorn U, Proud D, Lichtenskin LM, Kagey A, Norman P, Naclerio RM. Inhibition of mediator release in allergic rhinitis by pretreatment with topical glucocorticoids. N Engl J Med 1987; 316: 1506-10.

38. Chung KF, Dent G, Cusker M, Guinot P, Page CP, Barnes PJ. Effect of qinkgolide in antagonising skin and platelet responses to platelet activating factor in man. Lancet 1987; 1: 248-52.

39. Colombel JF, Cortot A, Neut C, Nomond C. Yoghurt with bifidobacterium longum reduces erythromycin-induced gastrointestinal effects. Lancet 1987; 2: 43.

40. Nubiola P, Badia JM, Sancho J, Gil MJ, Segura M, Sitges A. Blind evaluation of the effect of octreotide (SMS 201-995), a somatostatine analogue, on small-bowel fistula output. Lancet 1987; 2: 672-4.

41. Jack D, Thomas M, Skidmore JF. ranitidine and paracetamol metabolism. Lancet 1985; 2: 1067.

42. Dammann HG, Walter TA, Müller P, Simon B. night-time rioprostil versus ranitidine in duodenal ulcer healing. Lancet 1986; 2: 335- 6.

43. Grundy SM. comparison of monounsaturated fatty acids and carbohydrates for lowering plasma cholesterol. N Engl J Med 1986; 314: 745-8.

44. Yoshino G, Kazumi T, Inui A, Jusatani J, Yokomo K, Baba S. Probucol versus eptastatin in hypercholesterolaemic diabetics. Lancet 1986; 2: 740-1.

45. Geissler C, Hoston T. Double-blind trial of herbal slimming pill. Lancet 1986; 2: 461-2.

46. Skeith MS, Ana CA, Nicar MJ, Schiller LR, Fordtran JS. Gastrointestinal absorption of calcium from milk and calcium salts. N Engl J Med 1987; 317: 532-6.

47. Bals M, Knuth UA, Yoon YD, Nieschlag E. Transdermal substitution therapy for male hypogonadism. Lancet 1986; 2: 943-6.

48. Firth RG, Bell PM, Rizza R. Effects of tolazamide and exogeneous insulin on insulin action in patients with non-insulin-dependent diabetes mellitus. N Engl J Med 1986; 314: 1280-6.

49. Puddey IB, Beilin LJ, Vandongen R. Regular alcohol use raises blood pressure in treated hypertensive subjects. Lancet 1987; 1: 647- 51.

50. Nicholson AN, Pascoe PA, Spencer MB, Stone BM. Sleep after transmeridian flight. Lancet 1986; 2: 1206-8.

51. Cleophas TJM. A simple method for the estimation of interaction bias in crossover studies. J Clin Pharmacol 1990; 30: 1036-40.

52. Cleophas TJM. Carryover bias in clinical investigations. J Clin Pharmacol 1993; 33: 799-804.

53. Grieve AP. A bayesian analysis of the two- period crossover design for clinical trials. Biometrics 1985; 41: 979-90.

54. Sever PS, Pulter NR, Bulpitt CS. Double- blind crossover versus parallel-group in hypertension. Am Heart J 1989; 117: 735-9.

55. Mc Leod RS, Cohen Z, Taylor DW, Cullen JB. Single-patient randomised clinical trial. Lancet 1986; 1: 727-8.

56. Freeman PR. The performance of the two-stage analysis of two-treatment, two-period crossover trials. Stat Med 1989; 8: 1421- 32.

57. Woods JR, Williams JG, Tavel M. The two- period crossover design in medical research. Ann Int Med 1989; 110: 560-6.

58. Willan AR, Pater JL. Carryover and the two- period clinical trial. Biometrics 1986; 42: 593-9.

59. Fleiss JL. A critique of recent research on the two-treatment crossover design. Controll Clin Trials 1989; 10: 237-43.

60.Cleophas TJM. Interaction in crossover studies: a modified analysis with more sensitivity. J Clin Pharmacol 1993; 34: 236-41.
61.Senn S. Crossover trials in clinical research. Chicester:John Wiley & sons, 1993.

CHAPTER 8

CLINICAL TRIALS: NEW ENDPOINTS

Background. The Western community is currently increasingly involved in the problems of patients with chronic diseases. The wish to deal with such problems gives rise to new endpoints in medical research.

Results. (1) Priority will have to be given to subjective rather than objective endpoints. (2) Such endpoints will imply an ethical obligation to value palliation on a high priority rather than improvement of objective disease variables. (3) Such research can be done effectively only when investigators emphasize the human touch rather than scientific rigor. (4) In patients studied for chronic diseases dignity and respect for the aging have frequently a higher priority than the informed consent rule. (5) Such studies because of their subjective endpoints can benefit from specific designs that enable test-persons to express their own preference for one of the treatments being tested.

Conclusions. The focus of chronic diseases is on risk factors and symptomatic treatments rather than causation and cure. Priority is the patient as an individual rather than the disease. The issues of research addressing this increasingly important field have to account for such priorities.

8.1   Introduction

Etiology is based on causal thinking mainly. So is our concept of healing a disease. As prosperity grows and mean age does likewise, western community is increasingly involved in the problems of patients with chronic diseases. Nor do people usually die of it nor do they recover from it. Apparently the issues are essentially different here. Rather than the search for causalities or treatments that cure the focus is on risk factors, the treatment of symptoms, and palliation. These are elements that clinical investigators are not familiar with. Not too long ago palliative care was even denigrated by the scientific world as unscientific and more properly in the realm of nursing. So far, there is no gold standard for palliative care against which it can be judged. Obviously, we are talking of an underdeveloped aspect of medicine. Controlled clinical trials are the very instrument for quantifying clinical phenomena and treatment effects with substantial precision and account for the variations in a group of data. This is particularly so when endpoints are simple and objective and when strict criteria for the purpose of scientific rigor are used. However, treatments of chronic diseases address matters of rather subjective nature such as symptomatic improvement, personal comfort, sense of well-being rather than objective endpoints such as improvement of objective disease variables.

Also, the use of rigorous criteria may be difficult to sustain when evaluation of subjective endpoints require a more personal approach on the part of the investigators. The present paper takes issue with such priorities of patients with chronic diseases and is a preliminary effort for the development of an appropriate methodology of clinical trials for their assessment.

8.2   Subjective endpoints

Emphasis on human rather than technical effects of treatments is currently given some attention in the research of chronic diseases although quite modestly so far. *e.g.*, hypertension trials do currently focus not only on blood pressure but also on quality of life and symptomatic improvement. Unfortunately, practically all cancer trials are still having one single and most important endpoint, namely years of survival, no matter how miserable they can be once cancer has become manifest. The American Cancer Society has to be congratulated with its initiative to recommend cancer research groups to replace the so called "life years" by "quality adjusted life years" (Qualy's). However, this initiative is far from being implemented.

Quality of life is not a simple endpoint and rather ambitious. Also, it has roots in social and environmental sciences as well as biomedical sciences [1]. It is obviously for those reasons that clinical investigators have been traditionally reluctant to address this endpoint. In addition, a thorough quality of life assessment may have to consider items such as sense of well-being, functioning, physical symptoms, emotional status, cognitive status, physical performance. For a sensitive and validated estimation of each of these items questionnaires of at least 50 questions each may be required [2]. Such questionnaires impose a tiresome burden on patients, which may lead to unreliable answers [3]. An additional problem is that such questionnaires are mainly based on the investigators' interpretation of quality of life only and virtually never enable patients to rate the importance of their individual problems. The very best quality of life assessment will be the one that adjusts the data for the patients' very own ratings for quality of life. Such an assessment can hardly give a simple answer to the question whether one treatment is definitely better than the other. There is too much between-subject variability for that purpose. Rather the focus is on broad spectra of possibilities. Studies are not very conclusive and show mostly just trends, weak statistics, type I and II errors (finding a difference where there is none, and finding no difference where there is one, respectively). Yet the results of such studies will be important to our patients because even if they don't give a definite answer they will give an idea of the patients' real needs in a subtle and balanced way.

8.3   New ethical priorities

Research of chronic incurable diseases should focus on palliative care and quality of life, simply because it is ethical. Chronic diseases teach us how to look at ethical issues in a different way. Medical ethics has currently a problem with its very own identity.

Politicians think that the ethical obligation originates from "the freedom of the individual" and "human rights". To physicians who are involved in the problems of patients with chronic diseases ethics is based on the phenomenon of suffering rather than the freedom of treatment choice. Human beings have ethical value as far as they are capable of suffering. It is therefore an ethical obligation to value palliation on a high priority. Relative thinking does help to that end: do not try to live for ever, you won't succeed (George Bernard Shaw, 1856-1950) [4]. Palliative care is studied little so far. There is no gold standard for it against which it can be judged. Obviously, it is an underdeveloped aspect of medical research. Denial of symptomatic palliative care in practice is not uncommon, not even in patients with something dramatic as malignancy or AIDS [5]. Patients are generally treated by several doctors that act as a team which discusses every patient. So they say. However, actually, they don't. Instead, individual doctors have different approaches, and thus give different and conflicting information. Patients who are worried and hang on to every word that is said to them, don't know who is in charge. There is lack of continuity and what is worse, denial of palliative care. Such a denial is a shame on the medical profession. There is so much more that can be done. The scientific community must lead the way because it represents the brighest physicians of all and "noblesse oblige". What we need is controlled trials on symptomatic palliative care which must be signposts for the medical community at large.

8.4   Human touch rather than scientific rigor

Controlled clinical trials are experimental studies where investigators manipulate the treatment under study, *e.g.*, by using fixed doses and periods and many more strict criteria irrespective of the individual response of the subjects. Although this rigor makes it possible to draw stronger conclusions which is the very reason for using them in the first place, we may ask whether it is ethically justifiable to perform such trials with human subjects [6]. Humans ought not to be treated merely as means to an end: they must also be treated as ends in themselves. In trying to do so, we have to recognize a number of limitations of clinical trials. First, improvement of objective disease-variables may not be very relevant in studies of chronic diseases, as long as there is no improvement of quality of life or symptomatic relief. Second, a placebo is hardly in the best interests of a sick patient. It is definitely unethical with an established effective albeit not perfect treatment modality in hand. In this situation a new treatment should be tested against standard treatment. If this is not available is it ethical to use a placebo then. Maybe it's not, if we have strong arguments to believe that the new treatment is indeed better than placebo [7]. Such arguments are frequently the main reason for performing the trial in the first place. So, it may often be more appropriate to look for alternative solutions, for example, a self-controlled study design (using baseline data for control) or an observational study (using "outside controls"). A controlled clinical trial of symptomatic palliative treatment can be done effectively only when investigators are allowed to emphasize the human touch rather than scientific rigor. Those who treat patients with a chronic condition will experience that a more profound patient-doctor relationship is generally required than the one described by Griffith in his cookbook for GP's, entitled

"The five minute consult" [8]. In so doing, they will find out about particular aspects of patient-doctor relationships that are based on mutual trust and empathy on the part of the doctor. It may become quite intimate although sometimes in a peculiar way. Patient may also express themselves in a peculiar way by using stories as a metaphor rather than direct statements. Being receptive to such particular ways of expression as well as empathic ability on the part of the investigators may largely contribute to the success of a trial. Without a curative option, this may be even more so. In clinical trials, as opposed to regular patient care, patients are generally highly compliant and have a good feeling about the trial because they think it will provide something from which they can benefit. They also do not want to disappoint the investigators who have taken so much interest in them. These factors can influence apparent patient improvement with symptomatic treatments. Rather than viewing them as biases or placebo effects, it may be fruitful to identify and assess them and target them for systematic study [7].

8.5 Little emphasis on informed consent

Trials of chronic diseases are trials in which the informed consent rule is not so important, because in patients with chronic diseases emphasis on palliation, quality of life, dignity and respect for personal preferences on the part of the physician does have a higher priority than giving information about objective disease variables. The informed consent doctrine, thus, is a topic that needs to be reconsidered for the purpose of assessing the study of aspects of chronic diseases relevant to the patients. Moreover, although adopted as a law for physicians it does mean little to many chronically-ill patients. We know how easily they can give informed consent. Essentially, physicians' training and skill create an inequality in the physician-patient relationship that no informed consent can erase. Therefore, on the part of the physician it can never mean loss of responsibility. On the part of the patient it can never mean full responsibility. In elderly subjects dignity and respect for the aging frequently have a higher priority than the informed consent rule. If there is no curative option, this is even more true. Moreover, procedures for obtaining informed consent virtually never enlighten to the full extent the suffering due to side-effects and the subsequent risk of ending up even sicker than before. We should employ less aggressive life sustaining treatment for chronically-ill and aged patients simply out of respect for the natural course of life. The cost savings from such a reticent approach could then - in the current context of relative scarcity - be spent on patients awaiting care.

8.6 Self-controlled rather than parallel-group designs

So many unpredictable variables may play a role in clinical trials of medical treatments, that, by now, a trial without controls is becoming almost inconceivable. The following methods [9] are routinely used:

1) A single patient receives both a new treatment and a standard treatment or placebo (crossover or self-controlled design).
2) For every patient given a new treatment, a control patient is given a placebo or standard treatment (parallel-group design).

Weaknesses of self-controlled studies are (1) they can be used for purely symptomatic treatments only because if a patient is cured by a treatment he/she cannot be used again in the next period of the trial; (2) they require a relatively stable condition because if symptoms spontaneously improve results of a second treatment are biased. These weaknesses are unimportant when purely symptomatic treatments of incurable stable chronic diseases are addressed [10]. Instead, advantage can be taken of the strenghts of such designs. First, between-subject variability of symptoms may be large in chronic debilitating conditions and pain syndromes. A large between-subject variability reduces the statistical power of parallel-group studies and is eliminated by the use of a self-controlled design. Second, with a self-controlled design none of the patients has to use a placebo throughout the trial because treatments are crossed half-way. This is the reason that ethicists frequently do have less concern with self-controlled than with parallel-group designs. This point is particularly relevant to potentially life-threatening conditions. Third, a crossover design enables the test-persons to express directly their preference for one of the compounds being given. This point is less relevant for the study of objective variables, for example, blood pressure, temperature, blood flow. However, for the study of subjective variables, e.g., pain syndromes it provides valuable extra information.

Self-controlled studies are routinely used for phase I/II trials in which small groups are tested for short-term effects of new drugs. In phase III/IV trials the situation is different. Such trials are generally of longer duration than phase I/II studies. It follows that for the study of acute diseases that must be cured, only parallel group studies can be applied. Some statisticians and the FDA have even pointed out that in all phase III/IV trials a parallel group design should be applied and that there is basically no place for self-controlled/crossover designs here [11-17]. It may be relevant at this point to make a distinction between two different types of phase IV studies, (1) investigations among large numbers of patients in parallel groups issued for the detection of rare side effects of a new treatment rather than its efficacy (we exclude the so called promotional phase IV studies) and (2) large-scale trials for the purpose of the determination of the ultimate place of a new treatment compared to standard or placebo. Because common symptomatology is involved in the latter instance and not so much rare side-effects, this type of phase IV study could gain in statistical power by a crossover design, because between-subject variability of symptoms is eliminated. In addition, the costs of such research may be easier to contain because fewer test-subjects are needed and ethical committees will approve such trials more readily because seriously ill patients need not be treated with a placebo or an inefficient compound throughout the trial. One might contend, therefore, that for studying chronic diseases, for which treatment is directed primarily to relief of persistent symptoms phase III/IV crossover studies do have a place. All of the strengths are taken advantage of while the weaknesses are not relevant.

8.7 Conclusions

Clinical trials can benefit from a number of criteria: appropriate controls, scientific rigor including double-blinding, ethical approval including a written informed consent, simple and objective endpoints assessed by objective measurements, and a reproducible challenge test etc. The problems associated with patients with chronic diseases gives rise to fundamentally different endpoints: they are very complex and, in addition, almost entirely subjective. This urges the consideration of other criteria for these studies. It implies an ethical obligation to value palliation on a high priority rather than freedom of treatment choice. Such research can be done effectively only when investigators emphasize the human touch rather than scientific rigor. Also emphasis should be placed on dignity and respect for the aging rather than on the informed consent doctrine. A self-controlled design for such studies provides extra value in that it enables test-subjects to directly express their preference for one of the treatments being tested.

In conclusion, the focus of chronic diseases is on risk factors and symptomatic treatments rather than causation and cure. Priority is the patient as an individual rather than the disease. The issues of research addressing this increasingly important field have to take account of such priorities.

Acknowledgement

The author is indebted to the editor and publisher of Clinical Research And Regulatory Affairs for granting permission to use parts of a paper previously published in the journal (1995; 12: 273-82).

References

1. Wilson JB, Cleary PD. Linking clinical variables with health-related qualify of life. JAMA 1995; 273: 59-65.
2. Gill TM, Feinstein AR. A critical appraisal of the quality of life measurements. JAMA 1994; 272: 619-26.
3. Cleophas TJ, de Jong SJ, Niemeyer MG, Tavenier P, Zwinderman K, Kuyper A. Changes in life-style in men under sixty years of age before and after acute myocardial infarction: a case-control study. Angiology 1993; 44: 761-8.
4. Shaw GB. Mrs. Warren's profession. Oxford, UK, University Press, 1925.
5. Anonymous. The inhumanity and humanity of medicine. Dying for palliative care. Br Med J 1994; 309: 1696-9.
6. Cleophas TJ. The use of placebo controls. N Engl J Med 1995; 332: 61.
7. Cleophas TJ. The importance of placebo effects. JAMA 1995; 273: 283-4.
8. Griffith PL. The 5 minute consult. Philadelphia: Lea & Febinger, 1994.
9. Moses LE. Statistical concepts fundamental to investigations. N Engl J Med 1985; 312: 890-7.
10. Cleophas TJ. Clinical trials in chronic diseases. J Clin Pharmacol 1995; 35: 594-8.
11. Cornfield J, O'Neill RT. Minutes of the Food and Drug Administration Advisory Committee Meeting, June, 23, 1976.
12. Wallenstein S, Fisher AC. The analysis of the two-period repeated measurements crossover design with application to clinical trials. Biometrics 1977; 33: 261-9.
13. Zimmermann H, Rahlfs V. Testing hypotheses in the two-period change-over with binary data. Biom J 1978; 20: 133-41.

14.Hills M, Armitage P. The two-period crossover clinical trial. Br J Clin Pharmacol 1979; 8: 7-20.

15.Brown BW. The crossover experiment for clinical trials. Biometrics 1980; 36: 69-79.

16.Presscott RJ. The comparison of success rates in crossover trials in the presence of an order effect. Appl Stat 1981; 30: 9-15.

17.Barker M, Hew RJ, Huitson A, Poloniecki J. The two-period crossover trial. Bull Appl Stat 1982; 9: 67-112.

CHAPTER 9

LINEAR SCALE ASSESSMENT OF RELEVANT DOMAINS OF QUALITY OF LIFE

an example

Background. High dosage nitrates were more effective for the management of anginal symptoms, but produced more adverse effects, including development of tolerance and the zero-hour effect (rebound angina at the end of the dosing interval). Such effects may reduce the beneficial effect of treatment on quality of life.

Methods. In a self-controlled, 6-month study, the effects on symptoms and quality of life of once daily 50 mg and 100 mg sustained release (SR) isosorbidemononitrate (ISMN) were evaluated in 352 patients with stable angina pectoris. Quality of life (QOL) was assessed by a test battery based on the Short Form 36 questionnaire of Brazier and the APQLQ (Angina Pectoris Quality of Life Questionnaire) of Wilson. The internal consistency and reliability of the multi-item scales were estimated by Cronbach's alpha coefficients.

Results. Based on New York Heart Association (NYHA) angina classification, patients improved better on 100 mg than on 50 mg SR ISMN: mean difference of 0.52 (19.8%) between treatments (P < 0.001), consistent with a better improvement of both mobility and angina indices by no less than 20.4 and 13.9% (p < 0.001 and p < 0.001). Adverse effects as estimated by side effect index, including rebound angina at times of rest, and by compliance rating differed little between the two treatment regimens, and were, actually, slidely less a problem with the high than with the low dosage (2.9 and 2 % difference in favor of high dosage, p < 0.001 and p=0.006). Psychological distress index and life satisfaction scores likewise improved better on 100 mg than on 50 mg SR ISMN: differences 7.4 and 11.2-19.6%, p < 0.001 and p < 0.001 respectively).

Conclusions. Once daily 100mg SR ISMN preparation provided better NYHA angina classification than 50 mg SR ISMN, and did not produce more adverse effects.

In addition, and more importantly, 100 mg SR ISMN improved more substantially than 50 mg different QOL indices, particularly, mobility index and some life satisfaction scores, the most important indicators of quality of life in this category of patients.

9.1   Introduction

In our hands fifty milligrams of isosorbide mononitrate (ISMN) 30% immediate-release plus 70% sustained-release once daily performed better than multiple dose ISMN immediate-release in patients with stable angina pectoris: anginal symptoms decreased by approximately 20% and health-related quality of life (QOL) indices improved by approximately 5% [1]. In studies of others higher dosages were even more effective [3], but also produced more adverse effects including development of tolerance [4,5]. Also the risk of rebound angina at the end of the dosage interval must be considered with higher dosages, although it has so far been demonstrated with transdermal nitrate patches only [6,7], and could not be demonstrated in one ISMN study [8]. The present paper presents a completely new study of our group comparing 100 mg vs 50 mg ISMN in patients with stable angina pectoris. The study tries to test the hypothesis, that, despite the presumably increased risk of side effects, the net effect on QOL indices is in favor of the high dosage. This was considered to be probably so, because immobility and psychological distress due to immobility are more important indicators for QOL in such patients than physical symptoms including physical side effects of the medications given. The first objective of this study was to determine what would be the effects of the two treatments on physical symptoms, and adverse effects from the drugs given. Secondly, we assessed what would the effects on different health related QOL indices.

9.2   Patients and methods

Patients
This was an open label,sequential, multicenter, comparison of two treatment regimens of 3 months each with long-acting nitrates in patients with stable angina pectoris. Patients were sampled in 27 hospitals throughout the Netherlands. The admission criteria were: presence of coronary artery disease documented either by coronary arteriography and/or myocardial infarction or by clinical signs only; presence of symptoms of stable angina pectoris treated by beta-blockers and/or calcium-antagonists and/or short-acting sublingual nitrates ad libitum so far. The exclusion criteria were: insulin-dependent diabetes, the presence of serious diseases otherwise, hospitalization within 1 month prior to the study (especially for myocardial infarction, bypass surgery or coronary angioplasty); inadequate knowledge of language for self-administration of a questionnaire, major social problems complicating the medical condition, recent life events that might have affected the outcome of the present study.

Study design
Our study design was governed by the following statistical considerations:
1. Because this was a study of equivalent treatments, we considered it appropriate to include the possibility of testing not only differences but also equivalence of the treatment modalities [9]. For that purpose a very powerful treatment comparison is required. A parallel-group design seemed to be less suitable for such purpose because of the established large between-subject variability of symptoms in patients with angina pectoris, reducing the power of such an approach [10].
2. A self-controlled treatment comparison would provide adequate power. It was expected that treatments would improve different QOL indices by 5-10% [1]. Under the assumption of a baseline standard deviation of 25% and a between-period correlation of +0.6, at least 400 patients had to be included in the study to obtain a statistical power of 80% and a 5% significance level.

3. A crossover design would have enabled to perform randomization and blinding of the study. However, such design is endangered of physical and psychological carryover effects from the first into the second treatment period in the treatment group that receives the less effective treatment regimen after the more effective one [11]. It usually causes major underestimation of the treatment effect [12]. So, we decided to use a simple self-controlled design where all of the patients would receive the standard and presumably less effective treatment regimen prior to the more effective one. This design closely met the rest of our criteria including ethical and recruitment criteria. Moreover, self-controlled comparisons form a basis for many clinical trials [13].

All of the patients started on 50-60 mg ISMN sustained-release once daily (84% of them using 50 mg preparation 30% immediate-release and 70% sustained-release) which was standard therapy in the participating hospitals at that time, and all of them changed over to once-daily 100 mg ISMN 30% immediate/70% sustained-release after 3 months. The chance of time effects was minimized because patients with stable disease were included only. The chance of carryover effects was minimized because such effects are considered to be negligible when a less effective treatment regimen precedes a more effective one [13], and we had no basis for assuming that this was not true in our study.

Methods of evaluation
Patients were requested to complete a self-administered quality of life questionnaire twice, *i.e.*, after 3, and after 6 month treatment. On the same form the physician reported the actual patient characteristics: specific side effects of drugs given, the actual category of the New York Heart Association (NYHA) angina as well as heart failure classification, walking distance and duration of anginal attacks as estimated by the patient, and the level of compliance as estimated by the numbers of tablets returned and the patients' own rating of compliance, and the additional drugs used. The physicians also kept a register of patients who did not complete the study.

Questionnaires, additional questions
Various domains of quality of life were measured by a test battery based on the Short Form 36 questionnaire of Brazier *et al.* [14], and the APQLQ (Angina Pectoris Quality of Life Questionnaire) of Wilson [15]. In a self-administered patient questionnaire consisting of 31 items, we assessed 4 important areas of quality of life: (1) limitations of daily mobility, (2) anginal pain index, (3) side effect of treatment index, (4) feelings of anxiety and distress. In addition, we added three items assessing life satisfaction (1) with treatment, (2) with current disease stage, (3) with daily life pleasure. All of the items were scored on a five point ordinal scale ranging from "plenty" to "no" problems. Scale scores were calculated as the means of the item scores within the scale, and subsequently transformed (linearly) to a scale from 0 to 10 [16]. Lastly, patients were requested to estimate the extent to which they had forgotten to take their medication, and whether or not they had been taking short-acting sublingual nitrates during the past study period. The first and second quality of life questionnaire forms were identical except for an additional question in the second form on which patients could give their preference for multiple dose or once-daily nitrate therapy.

Statistical analysis

Patient and disease characteristics at baseline and after the 3 month and 6 month trial were analyzed with the paired Student's t-test, the Wilcoxon matched-pairs signed ranks test, or the McNemar test where appropriate. Although all of the indices used have been demonstrated to have a negligible within-subject test/retest variability in untreated subjects, we considered it matter of course to assess the internal consistency and reliability of the multi-items scales in our material. We did so by measuring internal consistency coefficient as estimated by Cronbach's alpha [17]. This coefficient represents the proportion of variance due to the true score as compared to the overall variance in the data including measurement error. It has a maximum value of 1 whereas a value above 0.7 is recommended to ensure acceptable reliability. A value of 0.05 or less was considered significant.

9.3   Results

The intention-to-treat population consisted of 398 patients: 35% females, 65% males, and none of unknown gender. In total, 47 (8.5%) patients did not complete the study: 20 were lost for follow-up and 27 needed more intensive therapy. There were no significant differences between the number of withdrawals in the first and the second period of the study. The efficacy population, thus, consisted of 352 patients. Their characteristics are summarized in Table I.

During the 100 mg ISMN period patients improved (on average) on the mobility scale (p < 0.001), had less side-effects, including rebound angina at times of rest (p < 0.001), less typical angina pain (p < 0.001), and had less psychological distress (p < 0.001). Patients also had more pleasure in their daily activities (p < 0.001), and were more satisfied with their treatment (p < 0.001). These data are summarized in Table II. As a result 83% of the patients preferred the 100 mg ISMN dosage treatment.

This improvement as reported by the patient was also recognized by the attending physicians (Table III). Angina class (NYHA) improved one or more categories in 44% of the patients, whereas it deteriorated in only 2.3% of the patients (p < 0.0001). Similarly, heart failure class (NYHA) improved one or more categories in 10.7% of the patients, whereas it deteriorated in 4.3% of the patients (p < 0.0001). This was not due to more beta-blocking use, which was used by 72% of the patients before, and by 73% of the patients after the switch of medication (p=0.58), nor by more calcium channel blocking medication (which declined from 55% to 53%, p=0.44).

9.4   Discussion

Based on NYHA angina classification, our patients with stable angina pectoris improved better on 100mg than on 50 mg sustained-release ISMN, a finding which was consistent with an improvement of both mobility and anginal pain indices by 20.4 and 13.9 %.

Table I. Patient characteristics (n=352)

Variable		
Female gender: (%)		35
Age (years): mean (SD)		69 (9)
Weight (kg): mean (SD)		77 (12)
Length (cm): mean (SD)		171 (8)
Smoking: (%)		13
Hypertension: (%)		27
Peripheral artery disease: (%)		27
Diabetes Mellitus: (%)		18
Hyperlipidaemia: (%)		53
Angina Class (NYHA): (%)	I	7
	II	32
	III	52
	IV	10
Decomposition Cordis class		
(NYHA): (%)	I	72
	II	17
	III	10
	IV	1
Beta-blocking medication: (%)		69
CCB medication: (%)		56

CCB = calcium channel blocking; NYHA = New York Heart
Association; n = sample size; SD = standard deviation.

Because this was a self-controlled study, it did not control for time effects due to spontaneous improvements. Although treatment with lipid-lowering drugs for several years reduced atheroma volume in patients with coronary artery disease [18], time effects within 3 months of follow-up are small as long as patients do not undergo revascularization [19]. Also, a placebo arm was not included in the study because we considered it less ethical to replace nitrate therapy with placebo in these symptomatic patients, even though improved survival with long-term nitrate therapy has not been unequivocally proven. However, placebo effects in patients with angina pectoris have been demonstrated to be more true in the physical symptom and side effect domains than in the mobility and life satisfaction domains [20,21]. Our data showed the most important changes in the latter rather than in the former categories. In addition, improved QOL reported by the patients was also recognized by the attending physicians who reported important improvements of clinical variables in the study group. The possibility of physician-biased observations was minimized by the use of standard quantitative questions rather than subjective estimates. These above considerations do not, therefore, support the presence of large placebo effects in our data.

In our previous study we demonstrated that 50 mg sustained release ISMN, 30% immediate and 70 % sustained-release formulation performed better than multiple dose ISMN immediate-release: it further reduced anginal symptoms by approximately 20%, and improved psychological distress and immobility indices of QOL by approximately 5% [1]. The current study of similar patients shows that a dosage of 100 mg ISMN instead of 50 mg of the compound once daily provides a 7.4-20.4 % further improvement of different QOL indices. Despite the high dosage, adverse effects as estimated by side effect index differed little between the two dosage regimens, and were, actually, slidely less a problem with the high than with the low dosage. This finding was unexpected. It has, however, been found by others as well [3]. Some of the socalled side effects, *e.g.*, dizziness and tiredness, may actually have been symptoms of the underlying cardiac condition rather than the expression of side effects of treatments given. Inportant adverse effects of high dosages of nitrates include the development of to-lerance and rebound angina at times of rest, otherwise called the zero hour effect [7,22]. The former effect did not occur in our study after 3 month 100 mg dosage since overall rating, rather than wearing off, became even more beneficial at that time. A question addressing rebound angina at times of rest was included in the side effect index, and revealed that rating of this item differed little, and was, equally unexpectedly, even somewhat better with the high dosage. In addition, and perhaps most importantly, mobility index and some scores of life satisfaction, the most important indicators for QOL in this category of patients [20,21,23].

Table II. Statistical analysis of quality of life after 3 month once daily 50 mg and after 3 month once daily 100 mg ISMN 30% immediate and 70% sustained-release formulation in patients with stable angina pectoris (n=352), as estimated by the self-administered questionnaire

	Cronbach α	50 mg ISMN once daily	100 mg ISMN once daily	% change between treatments	p value
mobility index score (SD)	0.90	2.20 (0.94)	2.65 (0.99)	20.4	< 0.001
side effect index score (SD)	0.89	3.45 (1.16)	3.55 (1.15)	2.9	< 0.001
psychological					
distress index (SD)	0.86	3.40 (1.19)	3.65 (1.15)	7.4	< 0.001
anginal pain index score (SD)	0.88	3.16 (1.03)	3.60 (1.01)	13.9	< 0.001
satisfaction					
with treatment (SD)		3.64 (0.98)	4.05 (0.86)	11.2	< 0.001
with current disease state (SD)		3.33 (1.04)	3.72 (1.05)	11.7	< 0.001
daily life pleasure (SD)		2.40 (1.20)	2.87 (1.29)	19.6	< 0.001

ISMN= isosorbide mononitrate

Table III. Statistical analysis of symptoms and patient compliance after 3 month once daily 50 mg and after 3 month once daily 100 mg ISMN 30% immediate and 70% sustained-release formulation in patients with stable angina pectoris (n=352), as estimated by the attending physicians

	50 mg ISMN once daily	100 mg ISMN once daily	% change between treatments	p value
painfree walking distance:				
median(range)	200m (2-400)	300m (2-5000)	50	< 0.0001
duration anginal attacks:				
mean (SD)	8.6 min (8.5)	7.1 min (5.8)	17.4	0.0034
NYHA angina classification :				
mean (SD)	2.62 (0.73)	2.10 (0.76)	19.8	< 0.001
NYHA heart failure classification:				
mean (SD)	1.39 (0.71)	1.31 (0.62)	5.8	0.005
patient compliance:				
mean (SD)	4.54 (0.80)	4.62 (0.74)	1.8	0.006

NYHA= New York Heart Association
ISMN= isosorbide mononitrate

Parker and Parker recently reviewed in their article in the New England Journal of Medicine [24] the current status of nitrate therapy and came to recommend (1) that slow-release nitrates, rather than beta-blockers or calcium channel blockers be given as an initial preventive therapy for stable angina pectoris, particularly in patients who respond well to sublingual nitroglycerin; (2) that beta-blockers or calcium channel blockers be given as initial therapy in patients with coexistent hypertension and/or a history of MI. We suggest that nitrates be routinely added in the latter category, given the apparent improvement of different QOL indices of such approach. We should add that nitrates are effective not only in patients with stable angina pectoris, but also in those with unstable angina, acute MI, and heart failure, although trials so far were not sufficient to prove a sustained risk reduction of MI or survival.

Quality of life assessments using problem oriented items only suffered from major placebo effects and were frequently negative due to lack of statistical power [28]. The current article shows that linear scale assessment of relevant domains of quality of life provides a more sensitive instrument to measure even small differences in the data. This is particularly so with paired comparisons. In the next chapter a slightly different approach to the assessment of quality of life will be demonstrated which may have a number of additional advantages, including the possibility to communicate more easily through odds ratios, extra sensitivity in case of small differences, and the possibility to easily adjust for confounding variables.

Acknowledgement

The author is indebted to Current Therapeutic Research for granting permisssion to use part of an article previously published in the journal (1998; 59: 511-9).

References

1. Niemeyer GG, Kleinjans HA, De Ree R, Zwinderman AH, Cleophas TJ, Van der Wall EE, on behalf of the Dutch Mononitrate Quality of Life Study Group. Comparison of multiple-dose and once-daily nitrate therapy in patients with stable angina pectoris. Curr Ther Res. 1996; 57: 927-936.
2. Thadani U, Maranda CR, Amsterdam E. Lack of pharmacologic tolerance and rebound angina pectoris during twice-daily therapy with iso-sorbide mononitrate. Ann Intern Med. 1994; 120: 353-359.
3. Chrysant SG, Glasser SP, Bittar N. Efficacy and safety of extended-release isosorbide mononitrate for stable effort angina pectoris. Am J Cardiol. 1993; 72: 1249-1256.
4. Kohli RS, Rodrigues EA, Kardash MM, Whittington JR, Raftery EB. Acute and sustained effects of isosorbide-5-mononitrate in stable angina pectoris. Am J Cardiol. 1986; 58: 727-731.
5. Thadani U, Prasad R, Hamilton SF. Usefulness of twice-daily isosorbide-5-mononitrate in preventing the development of tolerance in angina pectoris. Am J Cardiol. 1987; 60: 477-482.
6. Ferratini M, Pirelli S, Merlini P, Silva P, Pollavini G. Intermittant transdermal nitroglycerin monotherapy in stable exercise-induced angina: a comparison with a continuous schedule. Eur Heart J. 1989; 10: 998-1002.
7. Parker JO, Amies MH, Hawkinson RW. Intermittant transdermal nitrogycrin therapy in angina pectoris: clinically effective without tolerance or rebound: Minitran Efficacy Study Group. Circulation. 1995; 91: 1368-1374.
8. Olsson G, Allgen J, Amtorp O, Nijberg G, Parker JO. Absence of predose rebound phenomena with once daily 5-ISMN in a controlled-release formulation. Eur Heart J 1992; 93: 2052-2058.
9. Lee ML, Lusher JM. The problem of therapeutic equivalence with paired quallitative and quantitative data. Stat Med 1991; 10: 433-441.
10. Cleophas TJ, Tavenier P. Fundamental issues of choosing the right type of trial. Am J Ther. 1994; 1: 327-332.
11. Cleophas TJ. A simple analysis of crossover studies with one-group interaction. Int J Clin Pharmacol Ther. 1995; 32: 322-328.
12. Cleophas TJ. Underestimation of treatment effect in crossover trials. Angiology. 1990; 41: 673-679.
13. Louis TA, Lavori PW, Bailar JC, Polansky M. Crossover and self-controlled designs in clinical research. N Engl J Med. 1984; 310: 24-31.
14. Brazier JE, Harper R, Jones NM, O'Cathain A, Thomas KJ, Usherwood T, Westlake L. Validating the SF-36 health survey questionnaire: new outcome measure. Br Med J. 1992; 305: 160-164.
15. Wilson A, Wiklund I, Lahti T, Wahl M. A summary index for the assessment of quality of life in angina pectoris. J Clin Epidemiol. 1991; 44: 981-988.
16. Zwinderman AH, Response models with manifest predictors. In: Van der Linden W, Hambleton RK, eds Handbook of modern item response theory. Berlin :Springer Verlag; 1995: 175-195.
17. Bland JM, Altman DG. Statistics notes. Cronbach's alpha. Br Med J. 1997; 314: 572- 573.
18. Walldius G, Regnström J, Nilsson J. The probucol quantitative regression Swedish trial. Am J Cardiol. 1993; 71: 15-19.
19. Quyyami AA, Panza AA, Diodati JG. Prognostic implications of myocardial ischemia during daily life in low risk patients with coronary artery disease. J Am Coll Cardiol. 1993;21: 700-708.
20. Testa MA, Simonson DC. Assessment of quality-of-life outcomes. N Engl J Med. 1996; 334: 835-840.
21. Albert SM, Frank L, Murri R, Hyland ME, Apolone G, Leplége A. Defining and measuring quality of life. JAMA. 1998; 279: 429-431.
22. Demots H, Glasser SP. Intermittant transdermal nitrogycrin therapy in the treatment of chronic stable angina pectoris. J Am Coll Cardiol. 1989; 13: 786-795.
23. Marquis P, Fayol C, Joire JE. Clinical validation of life questionnaire in angina pectoris patients. Eur Heart J. 1995; 16: 1554-1560.
24. Parker JD, Parker JO. Nitrate therapy for stable angina pectoris. N Engl J Med 1998; 338: 520-531.

CHAPTER 10

ITEM RESPONSE MODELING AND QUALITY OF LIFE

We used item response theory (IRT) methods for the assessment of the psychometric properties of a quality of life (QOL) questionnaire used to measure the effect of two nitrate treament regimens in patients with stable angina pectoris. IRT methods have been used little so far according to Medline 1990-1996 in this area, but these methods can be valuable. QOL is a highly dimensional construct and is often assessed in homogeneous populations, both of which are direct threats to reliability which is mostly used to evaluate the psychometric properties of QOL questionnaires. IRT methods do not use reliability as a measure of their applicability, but instead use formal goodness of fit tests. An additional advantage is that the scale used does not need an interval nature. In the present application IRT methods were applied successfully and we conclude that IRT methods are valuable tools for in QOL research.

10.1 Introduction

Nitrates effectively control symptoms of angina pectoris, and reduce cardiac mortality at least in patients with acute myocardial infarction [1,2]. Following the GISSI-3 [3] and ISIS-4 [4] studies it is clear that they can also be safely used for long-term treatment. However, little is known about their effects on quality of life. This question is especially relevant because nitrates produce significant side effects such as headache, hypotension, reflex tachycardia, as well as tolerance if prolonged treatment is not discontinued for 8-10 hours daily [5].

In particular this last point brought us to hypothesize that a more effective dosing scheme would be more effective in controlling symptoms of angina pectoris, and consequently beneficially influence the quality of the patients' levels of daily life.

In the DUMQOL study we investigated the efficacy of fifty mg of isosorbide mononitrate (ISMN) in a once daily 30% immediate / 70% sustained-release preparation compared to conventional 3 times daily 10-20 mg ISMN or 50 mg daily immediate release isosorbide dinitrate (ISDN). Arguments for ISMN were as follows. ISMN provides better bioavailability than ISDN, because it has no first pass metabolism [6,7]. Sustained release was shown to have antianginal effect for at least 12 hours and may therefore be more effective in preventing drug tolerance [8-10]. Once-daily therapy is more convenient for patients, and should provide a better patient compliance, and the immediate release component protects patients from the circadian peak frequencies of angina pectoris early in the morning [11-12].

The first objective of the DUMQOL study was to determine whether this specific dosing scheme would improve angina pectoris in patients who were stable for at least three months while treated with 3 times daily 10-20 mg ISMN or ISDN immediate release. Secondly, we assessed what would be the effect on quality of life. In the present paper we report on this second question. We did not attempt to define quality of life, nor tried to measure quality of life in its entirety, but constructed a short and simple questionnaire assessing only aspects of quality of life relevant for the present investigation [13]. We used modern psychometric item response theory methods for the analysis of the questionnaire data.

10.2 Methods

Patients
Patients were sampled in 55 hospitals throughout the Netherlands. Inclusion criteria were: presence of coronary artery disease documented either by coronary arteriogram and/or myocardial infarction or by clinical signs, presence of symptoms of stable angina pectoris treated by beta-blockers and/or calcium antagonists and/or short-acting sublingual nitrates ad libitum. Exclusion criteria were: insulin-dependent diabetes mellitus, the presence of serious disease otherwise, hospitalization within 1 month prior to the study, inadequate fluency in dutch, and recent life events that might have affected the outcome of the present study.

Design
This was an open-label sequential self-controlled trial in which all patients started on 3 times daily 10-20 mg ISMN or ISDN immediate release which was the standard therapy in the participating hospitals. After three months patients changed over to once-daily 50 mg ISMN 30% immediate/70% sustained-release medication. Patients were requested to complete a self-administered questionnaire twice, i.e. after 3, and after 6 months treatment. In addition the physician reported actual patient characteristics: specific side-effects of drugs given, New York Heart Association (NYHA) angina classification, the presence and duration of early morning angina pectoris, and the need for additional sublingual nitrates. Patients rated their compliance, but in addition compliance was estimated by numbers of tablets returned and the additional drugs used.

Questionnaire
The life quality of patients with stable angina pectoris is mainly endangered due to limitations of daily mobility, pain, and psychological distress [14-19]. Therefore we constructed a questionnaire with a focus on these aspects. For daily mobility 8 items were included in the questionnaire assessing difficulties walking stairs, short and long distances, lifting, bending, light and heavy domestic tasks, and the profession. Pain was assessed by four items (headache, back pain, chest pain, pain in the upper extremities), and psychological distress was assessed by four items referring to sleeping problems, worrying, irritability, and sombreness. In addition three items were included assessing severity, duration, and frequency of anginal attacks between 8-10 hrs in the morning.

Items were scored on five points ordinal scales ranging from "no" to "very many" problems. Lastly, patients were requested to estimate the extent to which they had forgotten to take their medication, and whether they had been taking short-term sublingual nitrates. The two questionnaires were identical except for an additional question in the second form in which patients could indicate their preference for multiple or once-daily nitrate therapy.

Statistical Analysis

The item responses were analyzed by item response theory methods (IRT)[20]. The mobility, pain, early morning anginal pain, and distress scales at baseline were investigated with the polytomous Rasch model[21]. The goodness of fit of the Rasch model to each of the four scales was investigated using Glas' R-tests[22], and their reliability was estimated with the marginal intraclass correlation[23]. The response change from the first to the second completion of the questionnaire was investigated using the polytomous logistic latent trait model with relaxed assumptions [23,24]. This model is an extension of the Rasch model tailored to the analysis of repeated questionnaire data. The effect of treatment was quantified using the (log) odds ratio estimator which can be interpreted as the relative risk of scoring in category i versus i-1 given once-daily or conventional therapy. Effects of patient characteristics on item responses was also quantified using odds ratio's. IRT methods are well known in the social sciences, and sometimes referred to as modern psychometric methods. In life-quality research IRT methods have not been used much, but this is unjustified in our view. An advantage of IRT methods is that the analysis results can be reported in the form of odds ratio's which are well known in medicine, and which are (more or less) independent of both the scale used in the item format and the average population score. In addition different IRT models can be investigated and their fit compared, and the association with covariates can be estimated without attenuation due to lack of perfect reliability [25]. A p value of 0.05 or less was considered significant.

10.3   Results

The total sample consisted of 1350 patients: 848 males, 494 females (8 unknown gender). Age varied from 36 to 93 years with mean 68 and standard deviation (SD) 10. Coronary artery disease was affirmed by coronary arteriogram in 999 patients, and in 351 on clinical grounds. Additional patient characteristics are summarized in Table I. In total 138 patients (10%) did not complete the study: 51 were lost for follow up, and 87 needed more intensive therapy. Fifty patients (3.7%) died during the trial (31 due to cardiac reasons). There were no significant differences between numbers of withdrawals in the first and second periods of the study. As a consequence the effective sample consisted of 1212 patients.

Other than nitrates, medication did not change dramatically during the study. In the first period 53% of the patients used beta-blockers, 50% used calcium channel blockers, and 45% sublingual nitrates. In the second period these numbers were 55% (p=0.90), 50% (p=0.66), and 42% (p=0.06), respectively. Angina pectoris, however, improved

significantly (p < 0.0001) during once daily nitrate therapy: 281 patients (24%) improved
one or more categories in the NYHA classification, whereas 62 worsened one or more
categories.

Table I.   Patient characteristics

Male gender	848	(63%)
Age (year): mean (SD)	68	(10)
Length (cm): mean (SD)	170	(9)
Weight (kg): mean (SD)	76	(13)
Angina Class (NYHA) I	265	(20%)
II	849	(63%)
III	173	(13%)
IV	14	(1%)
Smoking (yes / no)	215	(16%)
Hyperlipidaemia (yes / no)	407	(30%)
Hypertension (yes / no)	400	(30%)
Diabetes Mellitus (yes / no)	143	(11%)
Arrhythmia (yes / no)	195	(14%)
Peripheral Vessel Disease (yes / no)	194	(14%)

NYHA = New York Heart association

In Table II the proportion of patients responding in the three highest categories
"some/sometimes", "many/much/often" or "very many/much/often" is reported for all
items in the questionnaire both after 3 and after 6 months of therapy. Early morning
anginal pain was quite rare in our sample with a prevalence of about 4% in our sample.
Pain and distress were more prevalent (10-20%), and mobility difficulties were reported
most often (about 30%).

The Rasch model appeared to fit excellently for the mobility, early morning anginal
pain, and distress scales with R_1 tests having values around their expectations (mobility:
$R_1=10.5$, df=7, p=0.16; anginal pain: $R_1=4.9$, df=2, p=0.09; distress: $R_1=6.2$, df=3,
p=0.10). The fit of the pain scale was less good (p < 0.001), mainly because of the chest
pain item. Removing this item from the pain scale resulted in an acceptable fit ($R_1=5.7$,
df=2, p=0.06). The reliabilities of the four scales were estimated as 0.67 (95% confidence interval (ci): 0.53-0.81), 0.55 (0.35-0.75), 0.88 (0.20-1.0), and 0.62 (0.44-0.80),
respectively. Chest pain was analyzed separately in the sequel.

The odds ratio estimates of once daily therapy on the quality of life aspects are reported
in Table III. Significant differences between the responses after three months of conventional therapy and after three months of the once-daily dosing scheme were observed
for mobility difficulties, chest pain, early morning anginal pain, psychological distress,
and medication compliance. The risk of (more severe) mobility difficulties was
(1-0.83)=17% lower under the once-daily dosing scheme than under conventional
therapy. Similarly, the risk of (severe) chest pain was 36% decreased, 35% for early
morning anginal pain, and 13% for psychological distress. Patient compliance was
much better under the once-daily dosing scheme. The (multivariate) effects of patient
characteristics on the item responses was quantified with log odds ratios and these are

reported in Table IV. The most important covariate of the QOL aspects was the NYHA angina class: the higher the angina class the larger the risk of mobility difficulties, pain, chest pain, anginal pain, and distress. In addition, the risk of mobility difficulties was increased in patients with diabetes mellitus, arrhythmia, and peripheral vascular disease. Patients using sublingual nitrates in addition to the regular nitrate medication reported more (severe) mobility difficulties, pain, chest pain, and distress. Female patients reported more (severe) mobility difficulties, pain, anginal pain, and distress. The risk of mobility difficulties increased with increasing age, but - in contrast - older patients reported less pain, anginal pain, and distress.

Table II. Numbers (percentages) of patients responding in the upper three categories out of five ("some / sometimes", "many / much / often", or "very many / much / often")

	after 3 months multiple dose therapy	after 3 months once-daily therapy
Nobility Difficulties		
walking stairs	429 (33%)	330 (29%)
short distances	354 (27%)	274 (23%)
long distances	587 (46%)	459 (41%)
lifting	464 (36%)	363 (32%)
bending	377 (29%)	338 (29%)
light household work	228 (18%)	194 (17%)
heavy household work	499 (42%)	421 (43%)
Profession	95 (15%)	66 (14%)
Pain		
headache	132 (10%)	126 (11%)
backpain	237 (18%)	220 (19%)
pain in upper extremities	258 (20%)	214 (18%)
chest pain	369 (27%)	288 (21%)
Early Morning Anginal		
Pain at wake	81 (6.1%)	52 (4.3%)
when washing	48 (3.6%)	36 (3.0%)
when dressing	55 (4.2%)	41 (3.5%)
Psychological Distress		
worrying	282 (21%)	222 (18%)
sleeping problems	332 (25%)	302 (25%)
sombreness	204 (15%)	168 (14%)
irritable	155 (12%)	129 (11%)
Forgetting medication ever	263 (20%)	195 (16%)
Sublingual nitrate use ever	692 (52%)	621 (52%)

When adjusted for the aforementioned effects the risk of mobility difficulties, pain, chest pain, anginal pain, and distress was not associated with once-daily nitrate therapy. Patient compliance, however, remained significantly better under once-daily nitrate therapy than under conventional therapy (Table IV).

Table III. Odds ratio estimates of once-daily nitrate therapy

	Odds Ratio (95% ci)		p
Mobility Difficulties	0.83	(0.76-0.91)	<0.001
Pain	0.99	(0.84-1.15)	0.85
Chest Pain	0.64	(0.48-0.84)	0.001
Early Morning Anginal Pain	0.65	(0.48-0.89)	0.006
Psychological Distress	0.87	(0.76-0.99)	0.036
Patient Compliance	1.92	(1.37-2.63)	<0.001
Sublingual Nitrate Use	0.94	(0.71-1.25)	0.68

ci = confidence interval

10.4   Discussion

We used item response theory (IRT) methods for the investigation of the psychometric properties of our QOL questionnaire. IRT methods have not been used much in QOL research. Looking in Medline 1990-1996 for the combination of the keywords "quality of life/QOL/life quality" and "item response theory/Rasch model" resulted in only one paper [30]. In our view IRT methods can be of great value in QOL research. Quality of Life is a highly multidimensional construct and is often investigated in homogeneous populations. Both aspects are direct threats to the reliability, as it is usually estimated in classical psychometric investigations of QOL questionnaires, because reliability is a direct function of the dimensionality of the item pool in the questionnaire, and of the variance of the true score in the population. IRT methods do not use reliability as a measure of their applicability, but instead use formal goodness of fit tests. Reliability can be estimated in IRT as well, but then suffers from the same faults as in classical psychometrics [23]. Another advantage of IRT methods is that the scale does not need to be of an interval nature. As a consequence, the effects of covariates can be reported *e.g.* with odds ratios, independently of both the item format and the population average [31]. This is of cardinal value if populations are investigated in which the prevalence of QOL difficulties is low: ceiling effects are much less a problem in IRT than with classical methods. In addition, odds ratios are well understood and much in use in the medical community, and results of QOL research are therefore much easier communicated through odds ratio's than using classical methods. For instance, "the odds ratio of (severe) mobility difficulties for once-daily nitrate therapy is 0.83 (p < 0.001)" is much better understood than "the mean mobility difficulties score decreased from 1.10 to 1.06 on a scale from 0 to 4 (p=0.007)". In the present investigation the fit of our scales was reasonable, except for the pain scale. The reliabilities were not very high, but this is to be expected with scales of 8, 4 or 3 items. Moreover, the incidence of mobility difficulties, pain, or distress in our sample was rather low. The lack of friendly software for IRT methods limits their applicability, but this is a temporary problem. For dichotomous items plenty software is commercially available (Egret [32], RSP [33], OPLM [34]), and for polytomous items such software is rapidly being developed. Until then anyone interested in applying the polytomous Rasch model to QOL research can obtain free software from the author. In our study three month treatment with once-daily 50mg ISMN 30% immediate/70% sustained-release decreased mobility difficulties, chest pain, early morning anginal pain, and psychological distress in patients with stable angina pectoris. In addition, patient compliance in taking the study medication was much better under once-daily nitrate therapy than under conventional therapy.

Table IV. Multivariate effects of patient characteristics on item responses (log odds ratios (geometric SD))

	Mobility Difficulties	Pain	Early Morning Anginal Pain	Psychological Distress	Chest Pain	Patient Compliance
Gender	1.39 (.13)[3]	1.30 (.17)[3]	1.24 (.43)[2]	1.13 (.17)[3]	0.32 (.27)	-0.10 (.37)
Age	0.014 (.005)[2]	-0.019 (.009)[1]	-0.042 (.021)[1]	-0.045 (.009)[3]	-0.013 (.014)	-0.009 (.017)
NYHA Angina Class	0.75 (.07)	0.44 (.11)[3]	1.67 (.25)[3]	0.64 (.10)[3]	1.57 (.20)[3]	-0.21 (.24)
Smoking	-0.12 (.17)	0.11 (.21)	1.11 (.64)	0.51 (.21)	-0.21 (.35)	0.76 (.44)
Hyperlipid aemia	-0.03 (.13)	0.14 (.17)	0.11 (.42)	0.26 (.18)	0.25 (.28)	0.04 (.37)
Hypertension	-0.50 (.15)	-0.33 (.17)	-0.18 (.47)	-0.59 (.19)[2]	-0.31 (.29)	0.23 (.38)
Diabetes Mellitus	0.34 (.15)[1]	0.05 (.24)	0.96 .49)[1]	0.31 (.26)	0.25 (.41)	0.05 (.57)
Arrhythmia	0.46 (.15)[1]	0.10 (.23)	0.56 (.44)	0.51 (.23)[1]	1.01 (.36)[2]	0.07 (.50)
Peripheral VesselDisease	1.04 (.14)[3]	0.35 (.21)	0.04 (.19)	0.42 (.23)	-0.01 (.35)	0.92 (.49)
Beta blocking Medication	-0.10 (.07)	-0.12 (.15)	0.24 (.37)	-0.06 (.15)	0.10 (.25)	0.51 (.33)
CCB Medication sublingual	0.17 (.11)	0.11 (.15)	0.50 (.32)	0.31 (.15)[1]	0.78 (.25)[2]	0.81 (.33)[1]
Nitrate Use Once Daily	0.42 (.10)[3]	0.48 (.14)[3]	-0.00 (.14)	0.49 (.14)3	0.85 (.23)[3]	-0.53 (.31)
Nitrate Therapy	0.04 (.05)	0.11 (.09)	0.05 (.20)	0.05 (.80)	-0.20 (.16)	-0.81 (.20)[3]

CCB = Calcium Channel Blocking
[1] p<0.05; [2] p<0.01; [3] p<0.001.

This was a self-controlled study and therefore time effects due to *e.g.* spontaneous improvement were not controlled. Lipid-lowering drugs and diet *e.g.* reduce atheroma volume[26], but such effects occur mostly after six months or much later, thus we expect little time effect in our study. No patient had revascularization in the study period. Another drawback of our study design was the lack of a placebo group. Large placebo effects can occur in QOL assessments [27], but mostly in the physical symptoms and pain domains, much less in the mobility and distress domains [28,29]. Our results show important mobility and distress stress improvements, and an unchanged general pain domain, and therefore we do not suspect large placebo effects in our material. In view of this we interpret the improvement of the QOL that we found under once-daily nitrate therapy to be real. The main reasons are a presumably better protection of the once-daily dosage from the development of tolerance, and better compliance. Consequently, the incidence and severity of early morning anginal pain decreased, and chest pain and mobility improved. As a result psychological distress was decreased as well, and as a consequence of all this, the physician observed an improvement of the NYHA angina class. We conclude that the validity of our QOL scales was good. The improvements of the mobility difficulties, chest pain, early morning anginal pain, and distress were accompanied by a similar improvement of the NYHA angina class. Similarly, the QOL scales were associated with the classical risk factors for coronary artery disease, and patients with more mobility difficulties, pain and distress more often took sub-lingual nitrates.

Acknowledgement

The author is indebted to W. Zuckschwerdt Publishers, München, Germany, for granting permission to use part of a chapter previously published in the book "What should a clinical pharmacologist know to start a clinical trial" (1998, chapter 7, pp 40-48).

References

1. Morris JL, Cowan JC. Nitrates in myocardial infarction: current perspective. Can J Cardiol 1995; 11S: 5-10B.
2. Jugdutt BJ. Nitrates in myocardial infarction, a review. Cardiovasc Drug Ther 1994; 8: 635-46.
3. Anonymous GISSI-3. Effects of isinopril and transdermal glyceryl trinitrate singly and together on 6-week mortality and ventricular function after acute myocardial infarction. Gruppo Italiano po lo Studio della Soppravivenza nell'infarto Miocardico. Lancet 1994; 343: 1115-22.
4. Anonymous. ISIS-4: a randomized factorial trial assessing captopril, oral mononitrate, and intravenous magnesium sulphate in 58,050 patients with suspected acute myocardial infarction. Fourth International Study of Infarct Survival. Lancet 1995; 345: 669-85.
5. Cleophas TJM, Niemeyer MG, Van der Wall EE, Van der Meulen J, on behalf of the ISMN study group. Nitrate-induced headache in patients with stable angina pectoris: beneficial effect of starting on a low dosage. Angiology 1996; 47: 825-35.
6. Abshagen U, Spörl-Radum S. First data on effects and pharmacokinetics of isosorbide- 5-mononitrate in normal man. Eur J Clin Pharmacol 1981; 19: 423-9.

7. Spörl-Radum S, Betzien G, Kaufmann B. Effects and pharmacokinetics of isosorbide dinitrate in normal man. Eur J Clin Pharmacol 1980; 18: 237-44.

8. Nijberg G, Carlens P, Lindström E. The effect of isosorbide-5-mononitrate (5-ISMN) Durules on exercise tolerance in patients with exertional angina pectoris. A placebo controlled study. Eur Heart J 1986; 7: 835- 42.

9. Parker JO, Wisenberg G. Antianginal effects of sustained release isosorbide -5- mononitrate (ISMN). Circulation (suppl II) 1989; 80: 267-8.

10. Nordlander R. Can nitrate tolerance be avoided with once daily administration of isosorbide-5-mononitrate 60 mg in Durules? Eur Heart J (Suppl) 1989; 10: 73-4.

11. Lemmer D, Scheidel B, Blume H, Becker HJ. Clinical chronopharmacology of oral sustained-release isosorbide-5-mononitrate in healthy subjects. Eur J Clin Pharmac 1991; 40: 71-5.

12. Scheidel B, Lenhard G, Blume H, Becker HJ, Lemmer D. Chronopharmacology of isosorbide- 5-mononitrate (immediate release, retard formulation) in healthy subjects. Eur J Clin Pharmacol (Suppl) 1989; 36: 177-8.

13. Marquis P, Fagol C, Joire JE. Clinical validation of a quality of life questionnaire in angina pectoris patients. Eur Heart J 1995; 16: 1554-60.

14. Taylor SH. Drug therapy and quality of life in angina pectoris. Am Heart J 1987; 114: 234-40.

15. Wenger NK, Mattson ME, Furberg DC et al. Assessment of quality of life in clinical trials of cardiovascular therapies. Am J Cardiol 1984; 54: 908-13.

16. Reeves JT. Medical management of the patient with angina pectoris: an overview of the problem. Circulation (Suppl II) 1982; 56: 3- 12.

17. Smith TW, Follicle MJ, Korr KS. Anger, Neuroticism, Type A behaviour and the experience of angina. Br J Med Psychol 1984; 57: 249-52.

18. Wiklund I, Herlitz J, Hjalmarson A. Quality of life five years after myocardial infarction. Eur Heart J 1989; 10: 464-72.

19. Mayou R (1973) The patient with angina: symptoms and disability. Postgrad Med J 1973; 49: 250-4.

20. Van der Linden WJ, Hambleton RK. Item response theory: brief history, common models, and extensions. In: WJ van der Linden, RK Hambleton (Eds.). Handbook of Modern Item Response Theory. New York: Springer, 1997, pp 1-28.

21. Rasch G. On general laws and the meaning of measurement in psychology. Proceedings of the IVth Berkeley Symposium on Mathematical Statistics and Probability. Berkeley (CA): University of California 1961; 4: 321-33.

22. Glas CAW. The derivation of some tests for the Rasch model from the multinomial distribution. Psychometrika 1988; 53: 525- 46.

23. Zwinderman AH. Response models with manifest predictors. In: WJ van der Linden, RK Hambleton (Eds.). Handbook of Modern Item Response Theory. New York: Springer, 1997, pp 245-57.

24. Fischer GH. Logistic latent trait models with linear constraints. Psychometrika 1983; 48: 3-26.

25. Zwinderman AH. A generalized Rasch model for manifest predictors. Psychometrika 1991; 56: 589-600.

26. Jukema JW, Bruschke AVG, van Boven AJ et al. Effects of lipid lowering by pravastatin on progression and regression of coronary artery disease in symptomatic mean with normal to moderately elevated serum cholesterol levels (REGRESS). Circulation 1995; 91: 2528-40.

27. Cleophas TJM, Van der Mey N, Van der Meulen J, Niemeyer MG. Quality of life before an during antihypertensive treatment: a comparative study of celiprolol and atenolol. Angiology 1996; 47: 1001-9.

28. Hunt S, Mckenna SP, McEwen J. The Nothingham Health profile users' manual. Manchester: Galen research and Consultancy, 1989.

29. Brazier JE, Harper B, Jones NMB, O'Cathain A, Thomas KJ, Userwood T, Westlake L. Validating the SF-36 health survey questionnaire: new outcome measure for primary care. BMJ 1992; 305: 160-4.

30. Kessler RC, Mroczek DK. Measuring the effects of medical interventions. Med Care 1995; 33: AS 109-19.

31. Fischer GH. Einführung in die theorie psychologischer tests. Bern: Hube, 1974.

32. Anonymous. Egret manual. Seattle: Statistics and Epidemiology Research Computing, 1991.

33. Glas CAW, Ellis J. Rasch Scaling Program (RSP). Groningen, the Netherlands: I.E.C. Programma, 1993.

34. Verhelst ND. One Parameter Logistic Model (OPLM). Arnhem, the Netherlands: CITO, 1993.

CHAPTER 11
IS SELECTIVE REPORTING OF WELL-DESIGNED CLINICAL RESEARCH UNETHICAL AS WELL AS UNSCIENTIFIC?

Compared with studies providing unremarkable results, studies providing highly significant results are more likely to be published. "Negative" studies generally receive less interest from different parties including authors, editors and sponsors, and so, not-to publish such studies is a common phenomenon. Opinions differ on whether or not this phenomenon introduces imprecision into the assessment of health research and care.

This paper gives arguments against and in favor of publishing "negative" trials, and tries to give suggestions for a more balanced approach to this problem.

Arguments against publishing "negative" trials include:
1. the real possibility of a "negative"trial being erroneously "negative";
2. the possibility that the favored treatment is, actually, inferior;
3. full-length reports of "negative" trials devaluate the quality of literature;
4. "negative" trials sometimes contain unimportant data;
5. "negative" trials contribute little to the accumulated body of evidence;
6. "negative" trials generally receive little interest and so, not-to publish them is more or less "natural".

Arguments in favor of publishing "negative" trials include:
1. no report reduces the flow of information;
2. it violates the promise to patient participants;
3. studies not confirming prior hypotheses are especially important;
4. any well-designed trial provides at least some evidence;
5. "negative" data balance against the overwhelming power of positive data readily accepted for publication;
6. not-publishing leads to unnecessary repetition of research.

Currently the progress of science is faster than ever, and so, new rules are required. Suggestions for a more balanced approach to the problem of selective reporting might consider:
1. careful planning before the trial begins, reduces the chance of biased and erroneously "negative" trials;
2. any trial, "positive" or "negative", provides probabilities rather than truths; this notion does not explain away publication bias, but it does make it less of a problem;
3. "negative" trials may not be appropriate for general journals but may be very relevant to specialist journals, as well as other organs of specialist groups;
4. ethic committees and trial review boards should address the issue of publishing as part of their function.

We conclude that properly executed trials should be routinely made available to the scientific community. However, we should not forget that clinical trials provide merely probabilities, and must consider a more philosophical attitude to clinical trials in terms of acceptance that scientific truths are rarely absolute.

11.1 Introduction

Compared to studies with unremarkable results, studies providing highly significant results are more likely to be selected for presentation at scientific meetings [1], more likely to appear in print [2], more likely to appear as full report [3], more likely to be published in widely read journals [4], and more likely to be cited in subsequent reports [5]. This phenomenon may introduce misleading conclusions about effectiveness of treatments and reduce the power of systemic reviews, and, consequently, introduce imprecision into the assessments of the progress of science. Opinions differ about the consequences to health research and care [6-8]. Some of us believe that trials are tentative, at best, rather proof of evidence, and that a single trial generally contributes little to the progress of science [6,9].

Selective reporting of "positive" data according to them would serve the shifting of unimportant data. This belief is challenged by others who think highly of well-designed trials, and believe that any trial, "positive" or "negative", is so worthwhile that it should be routinely published [10]. Single studies, for example, the CAST studies [11], PROMISE [12], PRIME II [13], "regression" trials [14] and many more current trials indeed contributed significantly to the progress of science.

In the present paper we summarize arguments both against and in favor of publishing "negative" clinical trials, and we try to give suggestions for a more balanced approach to this problem.

11.2 Arguments against reporting "negative" studies

11.2.1 ERRONEOUSLY "NEGATIVE" TRIALS

"Negative" trials may not be truly, but rather erroneously "negative", if they are under-powered. The problem is, that acceptance of the nullhypothesis of no difference is almost guaranteed by simply taking a small sample. Typically, the type II error will then be very large making the statement of being "negative" virtually meaningless. Erroneous trials need not be published.

11.2.2 AN INFERIOR TREATMENT MAY SOMETIMES MISTAKINGLY BE BELIEVED TO BE SUPERIOR

"Negative" studies may also be "negative" because an inferior treatment is mistakingly believed to be superior. However, from a statistical point of view this possibility is extremely unlikely [15]. Suppose in a study the mean result is +1 SD distant from the nullhypothesis $0 \pm$ SD. This means that we have to accept the nullhypothesis and the study is "negative". For testing the chance that our treatment is significantly inferior, a new nullhypothesis at -2 SDs distant from 0 is required. This new nullhypothesis is approximately 3 SDs distant from our mean result, which means that this chance is < 0.001. So, it seems that we need not publish a "negative" study out of worry that the favored treatment may actually be inferior.

11.2.3   FULL-LENGTH REPORTS OF "NEGATIVE"TRIALS DEVALUATE THE QUALITY OF THE LITERATURE

In medical literature there are already many "dull" articles, covering little ground for their length, and imposing a not so necessary burden on busy and jaded readers. The body of what is in the index medicus is generally considered to become rather worthless and of little interest within 10 years after the date of its publication. Much of it is so when it first appears [16]. Texts are frequently too ambitious, and filled with irrelevant details, and broad views, so that the main point is obscured, and both authors and readers easily get off target, and get lost. "Negative" trials are, indeed, frequently "dull" to a general readership. Publishing such studies at full-length further devaluates the quality as well as the readibility of the literature.

11.2.4   UNIMPORTANT DATA

Isaac Newton (1643-1727), founder of modern physics, was famously reluctant to publish. He was so, because he considered the body of his work not important enough to be published [17]. Currently, publications are the coins, academics must use to get through the tollgates on their way to academic promotion. Academics, such as Georg Struckhoff, of Kiel University, Kiel, Germany, routinely publish one or two papers each week. This pattern enhances the publication of unimportant data, and does not benefit science, or the community. The results of "negative" studies frequently consist of unimportant data. Publishing them generally does not substantially serve the progress of science nor utilitarian principles to mankind.

11.2.5   ANYONE TRIAL IS TENTATIVE

What medical journals publish is not received wisdom, but rather working papers.

No matter how important the conclusions of a study, they should usually be considered tentative, until a body of evidence accumulates pointing into the the same direction. Physicians know that clinical research rarely advances in one giant leap; instead, it progresses incrementally. For this reason the practice of medicine, as well as clinical research is inherently conservative. Physicians are reluctant to change their practices overnight for good reasons. "Negative" trials will contribute even lesser than "positive" trials to the accumulated body of evidence [18]. A single trial generally does not substantially serve the progress of knowledge, a "negative" one does even less so.

11.2.6 "NEGATIVE"TRIALS GENERALLY RECEIVE LESS INTEREST FROM DIFFERENT PARTIES

"Negative" trials generally receive less interest from different parties including authors, editors, and sponsors [18]. And so, it seems a more or less "natural" matter of course not to publish such data.

11.3 Arguments in favor of reporting "negative" trials

11.3.1 NO REPORT REDUCES THE FLOW OF INFORMATION

No report reduces the flow of information. It introduces misleading conclusions about effectiveness of treatments and reduces the power of systemic reviews, and, consequently, introduces imprecision into the assessments of health research and care.

11.3.2 NO REPORT VIOLATES THE PROMISE TO FUNDERS AND PATIENT PARTICIPANTS

Clinical research involves implied if not formal contracts on the part of the investigators, both with the funding bodies and with individual patients. Both parties assume that their involvement is contributing to a growth of knowledge. This implied contract is violated by investigators who, having conducted well-designed research, fail to make the results of their investigations publicly available. In addition, ethically it is hardly appropriate to allow patients the risk to experimental therapy, with its sometimes life-threatening side-effects, and then not report the results.

11.3.3 STUDIES THAT DO NOT CONFIRM PRIOR BELIEFS ARE ESPECIALLY IMPORTANT

Studies that do not confirm prior beliefs are especially important, because there may be something deeply wrong with these studies: either prior hypotheses may have been wrong, or the execution of the trial or the report itself may have been so.

11.3.4 TRIALS ARE CURRENTLY BETTER DESIGNED AND MORE POWERFUL AND PROVIDE BETTER EVIDENCE

Research literature is poorly organized, of poor quality and largely irrelevant to clinical practice, with often conflicting results from highly selected groups. This is partly due to poorly designed research in the past, subsequently giving rise to poor papers. Trials are currently better designed, and routinely include prior power analyses. In addition, research teams have at their disposal ethic committees, institutional and federal review boards, monitoring committees, national and international scientific organisations and physician investigators trained to comply with Helsinki's recommendations guiding physicians in biomedical research involving human subjects, to safeguard ethical and scientific issues [19] (Helsinki's recommendations are currently being rewritten to further improve such guidelines [20]). Research teams are, thus, better equipped today than they were in the past, to protect scientific objectivity, and the evidence coming from them, correspondingly, has more impact on the progess of science than it had before. All well-designed trials, that is, all trials meeting current standards as established for example in Helsinki's guidelines, whether they are small or not, "positive" or not, do contribute to knowledge.

11.3.5   PUBLICATION OF "NEGATIVE" DATA BALANCES AGAINST THE OVER WHELMING DATA FROM "POSITIVE" STUDIES

Publication of "negative" data balances against the data from "positive" studies that are are more likely to be readily accepted for publication [21]. This phenomenon led to overestimation of meta-analysis data and false-positive meta-analyses [7].

Obviously, without complete knowledge of all of the trials we won't be able to systematically evaluate treatments. Also, we won't be able to address, whether trials conducted are fair, equitable, and inclusive of all groups in society.

11.3.6   NOT PUBLISHING MAY LEAD TO UNNECESSARY REPITITION OF RESEARCH

Not publishing may lead to unnecessary repetition of research. Granting agencies will not know whether they are funding needlessly duplicated trials. They will also be unable to take a broader view, as to the direction of future trials.

11.4   How progress of science was made in the past

In the mid-fifties the dominant positivistic view on the progress of science was, that it proceded by a hyperrational process of strictly observational predictions from candidate theories that were then tested against observations in experimental settings. Observations were initially uncontrolled, until in 1948 the first randomized controlled trial was published [22].

Since then, the randomized controlled trial has entered an era of continuous improvement and has gradually become accepted as the most effective way of determining the relative efficacy and toxicity of a new therapy because it controls for placebo and time effects. However, trials were frequently poorly designed even so. For example, a consistent objection has been, that they frequently did not confirm prior hypotheses [23]. This phenomenon has been attributed to little power due to small samples, as well as inappropriate hypotheses based on biased prior trials. Additional flaws of controlled trials were recognized:
1. Carryover effects due to insufficient washout of previous treatments [24].
2. Time effects due to external factor such as the change of the seasons or to the natural history of conditions being studied [25].
3. Bias entering into the study because of asymmetry between treatment groups [26].
4. Lack of alertness of the investigators while taking histories, staging, record keeping, or the use of equipment that is out of adjustment [27].

5. Lack of power due to a negative correlation between treatment responses [28].

Any kind of bias was considered as potentially fatal to a study, and constant alerness as a prerequisite. In addition, without a mechanism to explain results, studies used to leave investigators with worries that results might have been due to bias of selection, detection or ascertainment [29].

It was generally believed, as the Austrian chemicist and Nobelprize-winner Rudolf Kuhn (1900-1970) used to express, that moves in scientific development did not involve rational choice based on comparative experimental succes, but rather something like community-wide "Gestalt" shift, in which whole ways of thinking, paradigms, were abandoned and replaced by new ones, a process ultimately converging upon the un-equivocal truth. Such considerations emphasized that trials were tentative rather then proof of evidence, and that they had to be confirmed.

In 1986 Williamson et al. [18] demonstrated in a review of 28 benchmark studies assessing the scientific adequacy of study designs, that widespread problems existed in the published clinical literature. They reported that according to their assessment criteria the mere fact that research reports were published in the most prestigious journals was no guarantee of their quality. They also reported, however, that after 1970 trials significantly better met the assessors' criteria than before.

11.5   Today the progress of science is faster than ever, and so, new rules are required

In the past few years a lot changed. Prior to approval, clinical trial protocols are currently routinely scrutinized by different organs, including ethic committees, institutional and federal review boards, national and international scientific organisations, and monitoring committees. Consequently, the chance of approval for poor designs today is small. Better quality of studies is also reflected in the above-mentioned review of Williamson et al., as well as in subsequent reviews on this matter [18,30-33]. Also the quality of reporting studies, considered inconsistent and generally poor before, is currently under scrutiny. In May 1998 editors of 70 journals have endorsed the Consolidated Standards of Reporting Trials (CONSORT) statement developed by JAMA, BMJ, Lancet and Annals of Internal Medicine in 1997 in an effort to standardize the way trials trials are reported with special emphasis on intention-to-treatment-principle in order to reduce treatment-related selection bias [34]. For investigators, reporting according to such standards will become much easier, and will perhaps even become a nonissue if all of the CONSORT requirements during planning and conduct of the trials to be qualified have been appropriately met.

Another important milestone is the initiative of the Unpublished Paper Amnesty Movement. In September 1997 the editors of nearly 100 international journals invited all investigators to submit their unpublished study data in the form of an unreported trial registration form. Submitted material will be routinely made available to the scientific world through listing the trial details on a web site, in addition to other ways as appropriate [35]. The International Committee of Medical Editors and the World Association of Medical Editors are currently helping these initiatives for example by standardizing the peer review system and training referees.

Standardizing clinical reports does not automatically secure that trials are free from bias and will not stop authors from misrepresenting how they conducted the trial and from exaggerating intervention efficacy as demonstrated by the usually higher proportion of statistically significant results in abstracts compared to the body of the study [36]. Although generally the progress of science will remain a slow process, there have recently been several examples where outstanding clinical trials gave rise to leaps in this process [11-14]. Against this backdrop many of us currently believe that all well- designed clinical trials, large or small, "positive" or "negative", contribute to knowledge. The position not to routinely publish or, at least, to make available of such materials, although such an approach may have served the shifting of unimportant data in the past, is no longer warranted in the current field of research based upon agreed multicenter protocols, informed consents, and otherwise of high-quality.

11.6   Suggestions for a more balanced approach to the problem of selective reporting

1. Proper methodology for randomized controlled trials requires careful planning before the trial begins. This planning must consider what the size of the trial ought to be for an important clinical therapeutic effect to be detected if it exists. The choice of size involves the statistical concepts of type I (finding a difference where there is none) and type II (finding no difference where there is one) errors (frequently referred to as α and β), the size of a clinically important effect of therapy (frequently called δ), as well as the level of correlation between treatment responses (frequently called ρ). Proper planning reduces the chance of erroneously "negative" results. Committing a socalled type III error (finding an inferior treatment to be superior) [15] might be avoided be accounting for the treatment that comes out most favorably regardless of statistical significance. The statistical chance for an actually inferior treatment to come out significantly superior is very small even in small trials as demonstrated above. So, even a trial that cannot reject the nullhypothesis of no difference, is generally able to reject the hypothesis that the new treatment is inferior to the standard treatment. It may be relevant in "negative" trials to consider more often the latter hypothesis as well.
2. Proper planning does not completely remove the possibility of difference by chance rather than true difference. A significant difference from placebo at p=0.03 means a 3 % chance of a type I error, and a 30% chance of a type II error. Any trial, "positive" or "negative", documents probabilities rather absolute truths. Although this notion does not explain away publication bias, it does make it less of a problem.
3. Negative trials may be "dull", and "dull" articles may not be interesting to readerships of general journals. However, they may at the same time be relevant to readerships of specialist journals or, at least, to other groups of investigators involved in similar research. For such purposes materials should be made available. Scientific meetings as well as initiatives such as the Unpublished Paper Amnesty Movement [36] may be helpful to that end. Unimportant data may not be rare in in-vitro and preclinical testing, it is currently rare in clinical trials, because if trials are valid, they must provide valid health research information. Although we should keep in mind that single trials generally

do not contribute much to the progress of science, we may accept today that they are not just tentative anymore when designed, validated, and executed according to current standards such as the CONSORT standards. Also we should not forget that the literature even now is full of flawed reports [18,30-33]. Flawed reports of excellent trials do not qualify for reporting. The issue of selective reporting should focus on quality criteria rather than results of trials.

4. The fact that negative studies received less interest [18] from different parties including investigators, readerships, and sponsors does not mean that we should not have an ethical obligation to make randomized controlled data available to those interested, even so, albeit few who, actually, are. If different parties are unwilling to report, ethic committees and institutional review boards may be willing to address the issue of publication as part of their function more often. Already some ethic committees require publication as ultimate proof of ethicity of the trial they approve [37].

11.7 Conclusions

1. Properly executed randomized controlled clinical trials should be routinely made available to the scientific community at large.

2. Clinical trials are important but not the only way of obtaining science. Preclinical studies, cohort studies assessing the likeliness of diagnoses and associations, diagnostic studies testing sensitivity and specificity of diagnostic procedures all provide major contributions to that end.

3. Considering that trials provide probabilities rather than truths and that bias is human, we must consider a more philosophical attitude to clinical trial results in terms of the acceptance that scientific truths are rarely absolute.

Acknowledgement

The author is indebted to the publisher and editor of the International Journal of Clinical Pharmacology and Therapeutics for granting permission to use parts of a paper published in the journal (1998; 36: accepted for publication).

References

1. Koren G, Graham K, Shear H, Einarson T. Bias against the null hypothesis: the reproductive hazards of cocaine. Lancet 1989; ii: 1440-2.
2. Scherer RW, Dickersin K, Langenberg P. Full publication of results initially presented in abstract. A meta-analysis. JAMA 1994; 272: 158-62.
3. Simes J. Publication bias:. the case for an international registry of clinical trials. J clin oncol 1986; 4: 1529-41.
4. Easterbrook PJ, Berlin JA, Gopalan R, Matthews Dr Publication bias in clinical research. Lancet 1991; 337: 867-72.
5. Götzsche PC. Reference bias in reports of drug trials. BMJK 1987; 295: 654-7.
6. Melker HE, Rosendaal FR, Vandenbroucke JP. Is publication bias a medical problem? [letter]. Lancet 1993; 342: 621.

7. Chalmers I. Publication bias [letter]. Lancet 1003; 342: 1116.
8. Egger M, Davey Smith G. Misleading meta- analysis. BMJ 1995; 310: 752-4.
9. Pearn J, Chalmers I, Vandenbroucke JP. Is selective reporting of well-designed clinical research ethical as well as scientific [letters] ? Dutch J Med 1996; 140: 220-1.
10. Cleophas TJ, Vandenbroucke JP. Is selective reporting of well-designed research ethical as well as scientific [letters] ? Dutch J Med 1996; 140: 509.
11. The cardiac Suppression Trial II (CAST II) Investigators. Effect of the antiarrhythmic agent moricizine on survival after myocardial infarction. N Engl J Med 1992; 327: 227-33.
12. Packer M, Carver JR, Rodeheffer RJ, Ivanhoe RJ, DiBianco R, Zeldis SM, Hendrix GH, Bommer WJ, Elkayam U, Kukin ML, Mallis GI, Sollano JA, Shannon J, Tandon PK, DeMets DL for the PROMISE Study Research Group. Effect of oral milrinone on mortality in severe chronic heart failure. N Engl J Med 1991; 325: 1468-75.
13. Hampton JR, on behalf of the PRIME II investigators. Randomised trial of inopamil versus placebo in patients with advanced/severe heart failure. Lancet 1997; 349: 971-7.
14. Scandinavian Simvastatin Survival Study Group. Randomised trial of cholesterol lowering in 4444 patients with coronary heart disease: the Scandinavian Simvastatin Survival Study (4S). Lancet 1994; 344: 1383- 9.
15. Powell-Tuck J, Macrae KD, Healey MJR, Lennard-Jones JE, Parkins RA. A defence of the small clinical trial. BMJ 1986; 292: 599-602.
16. Freiman JA, Chalmers TC, Smith H, Kuebler RR. The importance of the type II error and sample size in the design and interpretation of the randomized controlled trial: survey of 71 "negative" trials. In: Bailar JC, Mosteller F (eds) Medical Uses of Statistics. NEJM Books, Waltham, MA, 1986, pp 272-89.
17. Mill JS. Methods of scientific investigation. In: System of logic. London, Longmans Green and Co., 1865, pp 416-22.
18. Williamson JW, Goldschmidt PG, Colton T. The quality of medical literature: an analysis of validation assessments. In: Bailar JC, Mosteller F (eds) Medical Uses of Statistics. NEJM Books, Waltham, MA, 1986, pp 370-92.
19. World Medical Association. Declaration of Helsinki 1964, after revision adopted by the 41th World Medical Assembly, Hong Kong 1989.
20. Lasagna L. The powerful placebo. N Engl J Med 1998; 338: 1236-7.
21. Antman Em, Lau J, Kupelnick B, Mosteller F, Chalmers TC. A comparison of results of meta-analyses of randomized controlled trials and recommendations of clinical experts. JAMA 1992; 268: 240-8.
22. Medical Research Council. Streptomycin treatment of pulmonary tuberculosis. BMJ 1948; 2: 769-82.
23. Cornfield J. Recent methodological contributions to clinical trials. Am J Epidemiol 1976; 104: 408-21.
24. Cleophas TJ. Carryover biases in clinical pharmacology. Eur J Clin Chem/Clin Biochem 1993; 31: 803-9.
25. Cleophas TJ, Tavenier P. Fundamental issues of choosing the right type of trial. Am J Ther 1994; 1: 327-32.
26. Cleophas TJ, Van der Meulen J, Kalmansohn RB. Clinical trials: specific problems associated with the use of a placebo control group. Br J Clin Pharmacol 1997; 43: 219-21.
27. Moses LE. Statistical concepts fundamental to investigations. N Engl J Med 1985; 312: 890-7.
28. Cleophas TJ. Criticism of "negative" studies due to negative correlations. Eur J Clin Pharmacol 1996; 50: 1-6.
29. Cleophas TJ, Bailar JC. Statistical concepts fundamental to investigations [letter]. N Engl J Med 1985; 313: 1026.
30. Sonis J, Joines J. The quality of clinical trials. J Fam Pract 1994; 39: 225-35.
31. Moher D, Jadad AR, Tugwell P. Assessing the quality of randomized controlled trials: current issues and future directions. Int J Technol Assess Health Care 1996; 12: 195- 248.
32. Schulz KF, Chalmers I, Hayes RJ, Altman DG. Empirical evidence of bias: dimensions of methodological quality associated with estimates of treatment effects in controlled trials. JAMA 1995; 273: 408-12.
33. Cleophas TJ. Lack of real science of symtom- based care. Clin Res Reg Affairs 1996; 13: 167-79.
34. Moher D. CONSORT: an evolving tool to help improve the quality of reports of randomized controlled trials. JAMA 1998; 279: 1489-91.
35. Horton R. Medical editors trial amnesty: unreported trial registration form. Lancet 1997; 350: 756-7.
36. Meinert CL. Beyond CONSORT: need for improved reporting standards for clinical trials. JAMA 1998; 279: 1487-9.
37. Pearn J. Publication: an ethical imperative. BMJ 1995; 310: 1313-4.

CHAPTER 12
INFORMED CONSENT UNDER SCRUTINY, SUGGESTIONS FOR IMPROVEMENT

At the end of this centennial, as the 50th anniversary of the Nuremberg Code is commemorated, the consensus on individual autonomy and insistence on informed consent to research, that for the past 50 years has characterized bioethical thinking in human experimentation, is being scrutinized. Ethical difficulties with the informed consent principle include:

1. philosophically, a person's free "will" is a rather primitive and, essentially, negative human driving force;
2. neither on the part of the physicians nor on the part of the patients does informed consent respectively mean loss of responsibility or taking full responsibility;
3. informed consent is frequently less important to patients with chronic diseases and the elderly, because such groups have different priorities;
4. when it is realistic to believe that certain new treatments will lead to important progress, commitment to individual free "will" may be outweighed by the interest of the community. Ethical difficulties with the informed consent process include:

1. informed consent does not cover all of the major ethical questions involved in clinical research;
2. informed consent may be an obstacle to research when it causes enrollment difficulties;
3. informed consent may be inadequate sometimes and give rise to misleading promises;
4. the execution of the consent process may sometimes be too time- and cost-consuming an activity.

Consent information forms tend to create a positive attitude on the part of the participants, and do so by giving information of borderline adequacy. Suggestions for improvement of the consent information form would have to include:

1. Adequate information on both benefits and risks ;
2. emphasis on the testsubjects' responsibilities;
3. a rationale for randomization;
4. a note about the premise of the physician-patient relationship;
5. an educational note about the negative properties of free "will";
6. information about the hypotheses being tested;
7. information about ethical issues that are addressed through different routes;
8. disclosure about possible conflicts of interests.

We recommend that while there are additional ways to ensure the patients' best protection, the informed consent must stay, and should serve to inform patients and motivate them to participate in a trial on proper grounds.

12.1   Introduction

In 1945 an important step in the history of human experimentation was taken. The Nuremberg Code [1] was composed by bioscientists in reaction to the Nazi horrors. It requested an unconditional commitment to informed consent on the part of physicians involved in biomedical research on human subjects. The 1964 World Medical Association Declaration of Helsinki [2] went still further. We quote: "Despite consent the investigator remains responsible for the human subject "(rule 3); "Particular care should be taken to ensure that consent is not given under duress" (rule 10); "Whenever the testsubject is incapable of giving consent, a responsible relative should take his place" (rule 11). Today minor compromises in the consent process are increasingly being permitted [3]. For example, federal regulations in the U.S.A. now allow for the waiver of informed consent to research under certain life-threatening situations [4]. Also, phase III trials frequently fail to obtain a written informed consent [5]. After all, the consensus on autonomy as expressed in the Nuremberg Code did not prevent very recent research from bearly standing up to ethical scrutiny [6].

Is the consensus on autonomy which for the past 50 years or so has characterized bioethical thinking, splintering, and if so, what are the underlying mechanisms? At this time difficulties with unconditional commitment to the consent process are an obvious issue. Also, we have at our disposal additional means to protect the patients' best interest, and to protect at the same time scientific and ethical integrity of research. There may be circumstances where a standard consent process is flawed and counterproductive, and has to be improved. This paper tries to summarize ethical difficulties with the informed consent principle and process, and to provide suggestions for improvement.

12.2   Ethical difficulties with the informed consent principle

12.2.1   A PERSON'S FREE "WILL"

Modern philosophy contributed greatly to the conceptualization of ethical guidelines to human experimentation. The ethicist Immanuel Kant (1724-1804) [7] emphasized that human subjects should never be used as means to an end but rather as ends in themselves.

This statement strongly supports the idea of informed consent. However, the next generation of philosophers were not completely in agreement with Kant. Arthur Schopenhauer (1788-1860) [8] and John Henry Newman (1801-1890) [9], for example, concluded that a person's "will" is a rather primitive driving force, and definitely not the same as his/her best interest. Human "will" according to these philosophers can even be very negative and self-destructive unless agreed upon by notion as well as by the heart. "Will" can become a virtue only through such pathways, and reaches its summit when acting out of compassion with the "Mittmensch", rather than out of self-complacency. The consent process itself, however, does not take into account the possibility that a patient's free will may not serve his/her best interests at all in the first place. Also, it does not routinely weigh the potential interests of research to community.

12.2.2   INFORMED CONSENT DOES NOT MEAN TOO MUCH TO MANY

The informed consent doctrine although adapted in the many Western countries as a law exclusively intended for the medical profession does not have a legal development at all. Actually, physicians themselves invented it. It does not mean too much either. We know how easily patients can give informed consent [10], and we know that the patients' best protection is not informed consent, but rather the conscientious physician himself. This may be a paternalistic statement. One should not fail to appreciate, however, that physicians' training and skill - the reason after all that people consult them - creates an inequality in the physician-patient relationship that the informed consent regulation can not erase. The informed consent rule does nor mean loss of reponsibility for the human subject on the part of the physician, nor does it mean that the human subjects involved in a trial take full responsibility. These important ethical issues are not accounted for by the consent process.

12.2.3   INFORMED CONSENT IS UNIMPORTANT TO
SOME CATEGORIES OF PATIENTS

Informed consent is unimportant to patients with chronic diseases and to the elderly [11], because such groups have priorities different from the informed consent rule. They appreciate dignity, respect, and they would frequently rather have their spirits addressed than their bodies. Subjects suffering from chronic diseases teach us how to handle ethical issues better. Medical ethics currently has a problem with its very own identity. Administrators and politicians believe that the ethical obligation originates from issues such as "freedom of the individual" and "human rights". Physicians who are involved in the treatment of patients with chronic disease, for example, the American physician Loewy [12], do not agree and believe that ethics are based on the fight against suffering. Human beings have ethical value as far as they are capable of suffering. In such situations, it is, therefore, an ethical obligation to place a symptom-based, patient-centered approach on a higher priority than objective disease variables. This is not what trials usually do, however.

12.2.4   RESEARCH THAT WILL LEAD TO IMPORTANT PROGRESS

A commitment to protecting individuals may be outweighed by the interest of the community, particularly, when it is realistic to believe that certain new treatments will lead to important progress. Basically, research should not be legitimally carried out unless its importance to society is in proportion to the inherent risks to the subjects enrolled. However, the larger the potential gains, the larger the permitted risks. It would, of course, be a serious mistake to conclude that the interests of others in society provide a basis for limiting autonomy. However, even if we consider the voluntary consent of the subject an essential feature, this does not imply per se that we should make it absolute. We are entitled, even obligated, to undertake a weighing and balancing that analyzes the facts and circumstances of a particular case [13]. Quite specific harms to many may force us to contemplate exposing some to risks, so that all might be saved.

For example, trials that may solve major public health issues including therapeutic benefits for most people, albeit with a high risk for a few, are examples of such a particular case. Other trials may not benefit most people but just a few. These trials may, however, at the same time, give rise to smaller compromises of interests of enrollees. A risk/benefit approach to trials using basic utilitarian considerations may better serve both subjects and community than an unconditional insistence on voluntary consent.

12.3   Ethical problems with the informed consent process

12.3.1   INFORMED CONSENT DOES NOT COVER ALL OF THE ETHICAL ISSUES A TRIAL INVOLVES

Some major ethical issues in a trial are not covered by the consent process. Particularly, informed consent does not relieve the investigators from their responsibilities towards testsubjects nor towards society. Also, it does not cover more modern ethical questions such as those raised by the human genome project. Genetic manipulation not only involves subjects but also their families. A fragile concept such as voluntary consent does not stand up to the awesome power of research, the international nature of both medicine and disease, and the strength of the profit motive in health care. Competent institutional and federal review boards, national and international scientific organisations as well as independent ethical review and monitoring boards are needed. Even then trials will be performed that do not stand up to ethical scrutiny [6].

12.3.2   INFORMED CONSENT, SOMETIMES AN OBSTACLE TO THE PROGRESS OF RESEARCH

A problem of clinical trials is the fact that selected patients often refuse to give informed consent. The remaining sample may be small and unrepresentative, and its relevance to the patients' population at large becomes difficult to judge. If at the end of such laborious efforts, including recruitment of patients from different facilities, the results do not confirm the expectations of the investigators, one has to wonder if we should not explore alternative methods for the evaluation of new treatments including epidemiological evaluations that do not require informed consents [14].

One more, although less appropriate, way out of this problem, currently practiced, is performing specific research in non-Western societies, where obtaining informed consent frequently is far less a problem or where legislation does not require consent. This point is critical, for in the aftermath of AIDS, research in developing countries is directly relevant to a disease in developed countries. Some argue for the nonuniversality of the Nuremberg Code: it was invented for the western society only, and less so for third world populations with different cultures that are based upon sense of community and feeling of within-group solidarity rather than a tradition based on individual and political freedom and democracy. The West committed its share of crimes against humanity but it also provided means to expose crimes and produce reforms, and so it was included by people of all nations and races. It would, therefore, not be appropriate to tell the non-Westerns that informed consent regulations were not for them [15].

We would propose that informed consent is as valid in Africa, as it is in the West. Even more so because crimes against humanity such as sexual abuse, discrimination, corruption and abuse of power, are more commonplace there than in the West. After all, the informed consent in the West was invented as a defense from similar crimes against humanity.

As a matter of course, maintaining informed consent rules in non-Western societies does not relieve us from our responsibility to develop additional standards for protecting the participants' best interest and serving high ethical standards, similar to those developed in the West, including institutional and federal agencies to safeguard the ethical and scientific integrity of research.

12.3.3   MISLEADING PROMISES

Informed consent may be sometimes inadequate and raise misleading promises. It has, for example, been recognized [3] to be so in some phase I trials of drugs for cancer which used consent forms that presented misleading promises of cure. It is probably also true for many trials in developing countries in which subjects living in utmost scarcity are generally all too eager to give consent to a protocol, so convinced are they of its therapeutic benefits. Also inadequate, although in a different way, is informed consent in postmarketing promotional phase III-IV studies that generally does not address matters such as physicians' reimbursement by drug companies for enrolling patients as a way of encouraging them to prescribe their agent rather than a competitor's.

12.3.4   THE CONSENT PROCESS, A COSTLY ACTIVITY

It has also been recognized that an accurately executed consent process is a very demanding activity, in terms of consumption of both time and of money [16]. This is particularly so if one considers that obtaining informed consent is, essentially, more than obtaining the subjects' signatures. Investigators while obtaining consent have to consider the social, intellectual, and emotional limitations of the patients. They also have to make sure that prior information is appropriately understood, and that duress, either real or of psychological nature, is not involved. Efforts to such ends are time-consuming and funding these activities is generally expensive. In addition, these activities generally have to be funded within the trial budget, which means that it has to be at the expense of other costs budgetted in the study and that other quality standards that have to be met to execute the study properly, are at risk of being jeopardized.

12.4   Example of a flawed consent information form of a double-blind parallel-group study

In January 1998 the EFFECT Study Group (Effect duration of Candesartan versus Enalapril in patients with mild hypertension Trial) started enrollment of 350 subjects in a double-blind placebo-controlled 12 week parallel-group protocol [17]. The clinical study protocol had been approved by the ethic committees of the 19 participating centers throughout Europe. The steering committee has investigator audits every 3 months from the start and an independent monitoring committee has the mission to stop the trial when risks to the participants appear to be higher than predicted or when significant differences between treatment responses no longer justify to continue. The informed consent form is accompanied by three pages of patients' information which, in addition to technical information, contains a small section on possible risks (2 lines) and a substantial section on possible benefits (15 lines). The experimental nature is not addressed. We give some details:

Text   **Comment**

"The staff will tell you everything..."

Misleading promise

"Today new medicines with better effectiveness and fewer side effects are needed... Here is a new medicine, but it is at the same time very similar to other medicines currently tested..."

Informations of borderline adequacy

"Your treatment is at random..."

Explanation why so is missing

"4000 patients have already been treated, and were satisfied... All of them had little side effects... Risks are, thus, small..."

Informations of borderline adequacy

"There is no guarantee of improvement of your condition but there is a guarantee of careful watchkeeping..."

Improper motive for recruitment

"According to the procedures you will have to carry three times for 36 hours an ambulatory blood pressure device which measures your blood pressure every 20 minutes... Do not engage in heavy exercise or mental training, because it may not work properly, and the test may have to be repeated..."

Information on the unpleasantness of these procedures are missing

This consent information taken from a current double-blind intermational phase III hypertension trial shows how the informed consent procedure creates a positive attitude on the part of the participants, and does so by giving information of borderline adequacy.

12.5   Some suggestions for improvement of the informed consent procedure

Some suggestions for improvement of the informed consent procedure would include:

1. Routinely talking up the potential of the trial and talking down the risks must be avoided.

2. The responsibility of the testsubjects towards society must be explained. Also it must be explained that refusals reduce scientific reliability.

3. The reason for randomization must be explained: people have a right to know that they are involved in an objective experiment, the results of which are essentially unknown,but at the same time that their protection is safeguarded by competent physicians and a monitoring committee having the mission to stop the trial when patients' best protection is endangered. After all, in human experimentation the requirement of competency takes precedence over the desire for objectivity.

4. The informed consent should explain that enrollment in a trial does not change the basic premise of the physician-patient relationship. It should be stressed that participants should continue to address their physicians in the usual way asking their advise for any of their concerns.

5. Educational note about how negative "free will" sometimes turns out to be.

6. Informative note about the hypotheses that are, actually, being tested in the trial.

7. Informative note about additional ethical issues not addressed in the informed consent procedure but taken into account in the trial even so.

8. Disclosure about possible conflicts of interests, as routinely requested by scientific organisations and medical journals.

12.6   Conclusions

The informed consent form was invented as a defense against the exploitation of human subjects for economic or otherwise opportunistic aims of others. However, this was more critical at the time we did not have ethic committees, institutional and federal review boards, monitoring committees, national and international scientific organisations, and physician investigators routinely trained to comply with Helsinki's recommendations guiding physicians in biomedical research involving human subjects. At the end of this centennial the insistence on informed consent to clinical research is being scrutinized. It is obvious that the consent process has specific flaws, and is sometimes counterproductive to research. Admittedly, clinical research should provide efficient tools to protect the patients' best interests and informed consents have proven to be very efficient for such purposes so far. However, with the awesome power of research we are facing today, routine informed consents may not be good enough anymore to safeguard ethical issues involved in clinical research. Some would say that ethical committees and monitoring committees are better equipped to protect not only the scientific objectivity but also the patients' best interests than the informed consent process and that the latter is thus on the edge of becoming superfluous. This may be true in settings where all of the conditions to a proper trial according to current standards are met. However, frequently this is not the case and in such situations the informed consent still is a simple method to prevent major risks to the subjects.

Additionally, it is also an efficient method for providing important information to the subjects. We recommend that at this moment, while there may be additional ways to ensure the best patients' protection, the informed consent must stay, and that it should be used as a tool to provide patients with necessary information and motivate them to participate on proper grounds.

Acknowledgement

The author is indebted to the editor and publisher of Clinical Research And Regulatory Affairs for granting permission to use parts of a paper published in the journal (1998; 15: accepted for publication).

References

1. Levine RJ. Ethics and regulations of clinical research. 2nd ed. New Haven, Conn: Yale University Press, 1988.
2. The World Medical Association, Inc. World Medical Association Declaration of Helsinki, as amended by the 41st World Assembly Hong Kong, September 1989. Ferney- Voltaire, France, September 1989.
3. Rothman DJ. Book reviews, the ethics of research involving human subjects. N Engl J Med 1997; 336:882.
4. Adedeji OA. Informed consents in clinical trials. Br Med J 1993; 307: 1494-7.
5. Waldrom HA, Cookson RF. Avoiding the pit falls of sponsored multicentre research in general practice. Br Med J 1993; 307: 1331- 4.
6. Rothman KJ, Michels KB. The continuing unethical use of placebo. N Engl J Med 1994; 331: 394-8.
7. Kant I. Kritik der Urteilskraft. Leipzig: Dr Max Janecke, Verlagsbuchhandlung, 1920.
8. Schopenhauer A. Die Welt als Wille und Vorstellung. Berlin: Springer Verlag, 1819.
9. Newman JH. An essay in aid of a grammar of assent. Oxford, UK: Oxford University Press, 1870.
10. Cleophas TJ. Clinical trials in chronic diseases: new endpoints. Clin Research& Reg Affairs 1995; 12: 273-83.
11. Cleophas TJ. Lack of real science of symptom-based care of patients with chronic benign disease. Clin Research & Reg Affairs 1996; 13: 167-81.
12. Griffith PL. The 5 minute consult. Philadelphia: Lea & Febinger, 1994.
13. Christakis N. Ethical decisions made case by case. In: The ethics of research involving human subjects: facing the 21st century. Frederick, Md: University Publishing group, 1990, pp 434-45.
14. Cleophas TJ, Van der Meulen J, Kalmansohn RB. Clinical trials: specific problems associated with the use of control groups. Br J Clin Pharmacol 1997; 43: 219-221.
15. Hacker A. Research in non-Western societies. The NY Review of Books 1990; Nov 22: 64-5.
16. Cohen Stuart MH. Informed consent. Medisch Contact 1998; 53: 603.
17. EFFECT Study Group. Clinical study protocol study SH-AHM-0016. Saint Josephe Hospital Gouda, Netherlands, centre of coordination (Dr RP Hoogma), November 4, 1997.